Valerie Ann Worwood's

THE FRAGRANT PHARMACY

'An excellent encyclopedia for use in everyday life'
City Limits

'*The Fragrant Pharmacy* is a complete beauty and health care guide to
aromatherapy and essential oils, and offers lots of practical advice
on their uses in the home'
Woman's Realm

'Fascinating tips'
Cosmopolitan

'A lovely book full of details on the many uses to which essential
oils and aromatherapy can be put in everyday life . . . Excellent'
What's On

THE FRAGRANT MIND

'A definitive guide to using aromatherapy for all-round well-
being . . . A must-have for all aromatherapy fans'
Options

'Exhilarating . . . In fascinating detail, it charts how essential oils
actually take effect in the body, explores the mind–body link and its
untapped potential, and gives examples of aroma-psychology . . . I
think the words "monumental" and "fascinating" could safely be
applied to it'
Aromatherapy Quarterly

'This is the book aromatherapy has been waiting for. It provides a
wealth of new information on the human mind as it responds to
essential oils, with reference both to mental health and personality.
At 500 pages *The Fragrant Mind* is another magnum opus in the
library of aromatherapy and its implications are, perhaps, even more
important than those of Worwood's *The Fragrant Pharmacy* . . . Very
informative, comprehensive and practical'
Aromatherapy Times

'If you want accurate, detailed information backed by research and
experience, this is the book for you'
Here's Health

*Also by Valerie Ann Worwood and published by
Bantam Books*

THE FRAGRANT PHARMACY
THE FRAGRANT MIND

FRAGRANT SENSUALITY

Aromantics and Nature's Essential Oils

Valerie Ann Worwood

BANTAM BOOKS
TORONTO · NEW YORK · LONDON · SYDNEY · AUCKLAND

FRAGRANT SENSUALITY
A BANTAM BOOK : 0 553 50499 1

Originally published in Great Britain as *Aromantics* by Pan Books
Ltd.

PRINTING HISTORY
Pan Books edition published 1987
Bantam Books revised edition published 1993
Bantam edition reprinted 1995
Bantam edition reissued as *Fragrant Sensuality* 1996

Set in 11/12pt Linotype Palatino by
Chippendale Type Ltd, Otley, West Yorkshire.

Bantam Books are published by Transworld Publishers Ltd,
61–63 Uxbridge Road, Ealing, London W5 5SA,
in Australia by Transworld Publishers (Australia) Pty Ltd,
15–25 Helles Avenue, Moorebank, NSW 2170,
and in New Zealand by Transworld Publishers (NZ) Ltd,
3 William Pickering Drive, Albany, Auckland.

Printed and bound in Great Britain by
Cox & Wyman Ltd, Reading, Berkshire.

I wish to dedicate this book to my daughter, Emma Daisy, and my Aromantic friends who have filled my life with fragrance and beauty. To the unseen hands that gently and patiently guide and protect us all, may I say thank you.

A Special Thank You

A sincere thank you goes to sexologist Julia Stonehouse
for sharing her invaluable knowledge and contributing
specialist research. Julia's encouragement in the face of
adversity helped me to realize this book, and the
importance of using the written word to reach many
people, instead of lecturing to a chosen few. I never
truly appreciated just how many lives would be
touched and how many could be helped in this way.
Julia is a truly fragrant soul.

Contents

Introduction

'The most beautiful thing we can experience is the mysterious. It is the source of all true science.'

ALBERT EINSTEIN

Introduction

Like lovers, the jasmine flower responds to the moon. When the stars are shining bright on a warm summer's night and the moon is uppermost, the essential oil of jasmine is drawn inexorably upwards so that it's concentrated on the outer edge of the petals – which quiver, happy, like lovers in an embrace. Jasmine's perfume exudes, tempting her lovers into the perfumed garden to share her delight.

Love puts zest into our lives and zest puts life into the citrus fruit! Peel an orange to release its essential oil – the 'zest' from the rind that spurts out and stings your eye. But love can be dangerous, and nature can be too. In southern Europe the Diptan tree exudes so much essential oil its leaves can be set alight by a single match. Just one thoughtless move can destroy an entire forest as easily as it can destroy a human heart.

Fragrant Sensuality is about nature and romance. It's about attracting a particular sexual partner by using blends of nature's essential oils. It's about relaxation and excitation, well-being and self-confidence, and creating a balance of body and mind. *Fragrant Sensuality* is about sensuality and, yes, sex.

We shall see what the essential oils are, and learn about the mysterious sense of smell and how molecules of aroma directly involve our emotion and memory, affecting the way we respond to someone else. We shall examine the eight processes by which nature's essential oils work through the body-mind as aphrodisiacs. And you will learn how to release your vibrant Aromantic self.

The essential oils come from many different parts of nature's plant life. They come from the rind of fruit, from leaves, petals, flowering tops, seeds, roots and underground stems, bark and wood. Some plant species produce more than one oil from more than one part.

There could be over a million botanical species in the world – we're still counting them up – but not all are used in the production of essential oils. Nevertheless, we still use quite a few. In Europe alone five hundred plants are utilized, and although the majority of these are indigenous to small corners of the continent, many are widely used and exported throughout the whole world.

Indeed, wherever you go you can be sure that an essential oil has passed the same way. If they had ports in Paraguay they'd be packing pettigraine; in Zanzibar, it's clove. Come back from Bulgaria with otto of rose, and return from Russia with pine. Take the aeroplane to America for peppermint; the ferry to France for lavender; and the slow boat to China for aniseed. You name the country, there's an essential oil being produced there that someone on the other side of the world wants to buy.

This trade is not only widespread, but ancient. Today the petroleum oil trade is crucial and a cause of worry and war, but in times past it was the essential oils of nature that caused fleets to sail and armies to fight. For example, a Babylonian clay tablet details an order for 'oil of cedar, myrrh, and cypress to be obtained from abroad'. Herodotus records that in 600BC the Arabians were expected to furnish the war-like Assyrians with one thousand talents of frankincense each year.

Over three thousand years ago the Egyptian bodies

we see in our museums were embalmed in resins and essential oils which the aromatherapist still uses today. The mummy-embalming process wasn't about covering up bad smells, but about actually preventing putrefaction – and the ancient flesh is still there to prove that it worked.

For thousands of years humanity has used nature's essential oils to reinforce life. They and the plants they are derived from were once humanity's only form of medicine, and today they still provide the active ingredients for many modern drugs. Technology has only confirmed the empirical knowledge of our ancestors and proved that nature has provided us with a miscellany of oils to match a miscellany of human needs – and that includes the need for healthy, happy sex. Of course, nature's primary concern is for reproduction and, as you would expect, she has her means for encouraging this. Certainly, in the past people have thought so. A perfect example occurs in the classic Indian poem, the *Ritusanhara*:

> 'With their soft hips covered with beautiful fabrics and wrappings, their breasts perfumed with sandalwood, covered with necklaces and jewels, and with hair perfumed from the bath, the beautiful women coax their lovers to burning desire.'

In *Fragrant Sensuality*, for the first time, you will find all the information you need to potentize your life with nature's powerful and precious crop. The essential oils are about enhancing the positive, and fulfilling potential. You will learn how the oils work through the body and mind to release an inner vibrancy and harmony that is unmistakable and irresistible. There are hundreds of oils and dozens of ways of using them, and in *Fragrant Sensuality* you can follow my exclusive formulas or learn how to tailor-make your own – for you and your lover. *Fragrant Sensuality* is about exploration, enjoyment, health, happiness, fun and ecstasy, so prepare to be taken on a luxurious adventure where you will discover the new, Aromantic you!

1

What Are Nature's Essential Oils?

The most obvious thing about nature's essential oils is that they smell divine. This could lead you to assume that they're just perfume – sweet-smelling substances which make our lives more pleasurable. This is, of course, true, but it's only the beginning.

Essential oils are extremely complex substances which are rich in energy. They are produced by certain varieties of plant life and, depending on the variety, are stored in the petals, or the leaves, stalks, seeds, roots, wood or bark. They come from the tiniest flowers and from the highest trees. In some, different oils come from different parts of the plant. All the essential oils are unique, and their chemical complexity baffles scientists.

In 1980 Dr Taylor, ex-University of Austin, Texas, was quoted as saying that essential oils 'present more new compounds than the chemists of the whole world could analyse in a thousand years'. That was probably an overstatement in view of ever more sophisticated methods of analysis, but it will still be some time before science can give us the definitive explanation of what, exactly, they are. We know they contain terpenes, alcohols, esters, aldehydes, ketones and phenols, but some essential oils contain over a hundred compounds and isolating them all is not easy. The gas chromatograph can separate out some components by looking at the 'chemical fingerprint' produced, but there are unknown compounds, too, and it's useless having a fingerprint when you don't know who or what it belongs to because their details aren't 'on file'!

Essential oils are chemically very heterogeneous, and very diverse in their effects. This gives them a paradoxical nature which can be difficult to grasp until we compare them to another group of nature which is also apparently paradoxical – human beings! For example, one woman can be an accountant during the working week, a violinist in her spare time, a volunteer with the local paramedical group on alternate weekends, a charity worker on an occasional basis and a mother of three at all times! She's capable of many roles, and so too are nature's essential oils. For example, the same bottle of rosemary oil could be used to treat rheumatism in your grandma, sinusitis in your husband and acne in your teenager.

Plants in general are chemical factories. They inhabit the interface between light and dark, sun and earth, taking energy from both and synthesizing it into molecules of carbohydrates, proteins and fats. These are the 'crude fuels' which we, the walking chemical factories, break down to produce ATP, our 'high grade fuel'.

Certainly the human organism has an affinity with nature's essential oils, which absorb into and pass through the body with great ease. Many scientific experiments have shown the relative speed with which the oils penetrate the skin when applied through massage or osmosis (water) (Strahli, Katz, Rommelt, et al.) The molecules of essential oils are absolutely tiny and can penetrate the fatty layers of the skin into the interstitial fluid (which surrounds all body cells), the bloodstream and the lymph system. Also, those essential oils with smaller molecules may travel transcellularly, i.e., directly through the cell. The lipid solubility of certain essential oils may also be a factor in their penetrative ability. One hypothesis is that because the essential oils are not soluble in water their ability to penetrate is related to the fact that water constitutes so much of our organism. The human male's weight is 60 per cent body fluids, the woman's is 50 per cent and the child's 65 per cent. About 55 per cent of a person's body fluid is contained within the cell; the lymph and interstitial fluid account for 20 per cent; the blood plasma, 7.5 per cent; bone water, 7.5 per cent; connective tissue water, 7.5 per cent; and the cerebrospinal fluid and eyes and ears account for the last 2.5 per cent. It's important to realize too, that the essential oils are soluble in fats, of which, of course, we are also made.

Dr Schilcher of Frien University, Berlin, found that the essential oils enter the bloodstream quicker by inhalation than by oral application. Indeed, oral application has been found to be the least effective method of use. Their high electrical resistance means they are non-invasive to the body in the heat, electrical and magnetic senses, in addition to their usual non-invasive chemical sense.

All the above faculties mean that essential oils can easily connect with the area which needs realignment and healing. This has not gone unnoticed by the pharmaceutical industry, which hopes to harness the energy of the essential oils as a delivery system for its chemical drugs.

Millennia before people needed 'scientific proof' of a thing before they would believe in it, the essential oils were being extracted for medicinal purposes. Indeed, the aromatic plants of the world are humanity's oldest and dearest friends. Sixty thousand years ago in Iraq, yarrow, groundsel and grape hyacinth were used, possibly for medicinal purposes – as they are used today in the same region. In caves in southern France which were inhabited 30,000 years ago, juniper was burnt in the fires – and not just for heat. The oldest-known medicinal oil was perhaps that extracted from the neem tree of India. Many parts of the tree itself have been used since at least 4000BC, and the spiritual association made with it is clear from the Harappan seals of the Indus Valley civilization. In 550BC the 'father of medicine', Hippocrates, classed essential oils as medicines. When everyone was dropping like ninepins during London's great plague in 1665, the only group of people not affected were those working in the perfume houses which, in those days of course, used only the natural essential oils. And the spice wars of history weren't just about gourmands adding spice to their food or perfume to their powdered wigs, but about people trying to get hold of the raw materials that would prevent them dying.

Each essential oil has its own medicinal properties; indeed, *several*. These have been proven over many years by practical application and, more recently, by scientific research. Those properties also include (to name but a few) bactericidal, anti-viral, anti-toxic, anti-neuralgic, diuretic, anti-rheumatic, anti-spasmodic and anti-venomous. In a review of scientific literature, Dr Schilcher of the Frien University in Berlin reported that the particular oils studied have, among others, hyperaemic, anti-inflammatory, antiseptic/disinfectant, granulation-stimulating, deodorizing, expectorating, and circulation-stimulating qualities. Many doctors, especially in western and eastern Europe, use them to treat every kind of medical condition, including cancerous wounds, gangrenous wounds, skin diseases, burns, bronchitis and glandular imbalances.

You're probably wondering by now, if they're so effective, why you have never heard of them before. And the answer is that you're probably using them already, because about one third of modern drugs are based on them. But you wouldn't recognize them unless you looked them up in the medical dictionary, because they are hidden behind long, impressive names. But what is more impressive is their effect. Scientists have taken the typhoid bacillus and knocked it dead with cinnamon oil in twelve minutes. Clove took

8

twenty-five minutes, while Indian verbena and geranium took a little longer at under fifty minutes. And there's plenty of work on bacteria by other respected scientists that shows equally impressive results. For example, as an antiseptic, oil of thyme is twelve times more effective than carbolic acid, but in a technologically arrogant age 'carbolic acid' sounds more efficient than 'thyme'.

The essential oils leave the body as peacefully and easily as they enter. Depending on the particular oil, they take the usual routes of excretion: urine, faeces, perspiration and exhalation from the lungs. Indeed, the essential oils are extremely effective in eradicating from the body all sorts of dangerous toxins, including heavy metals, free radicals and viruses.

In the human body, balance is everything. For example, only 1 per cent of the calcium in the body is 'free roaming', while the other 99 per cent makes up the bones and teeth. Yet this 1 per cent is vitally important to blood coagulation, controlling the permeability of the membranes – especially of the nervous system, and the action of the heart and muscle. Oxygen needs to be kept at a balance, as does the pH value, the activity of the enzymes and amino acids, amongst others. The essential oils are, perhaps above all, natural balancers. They have the ability to effect changes in many different areas – maintaining the balance between oxidation and reduction, and because their pH value is usually acid, discouraging the proliferation of microbes.

The oils are, indeed, about checks and balances. According to Dr Jean Valnet, 'the high resistance of essences . . . discourages the diffusion of infections and toxins'. Their well-known painkiller effect with, for example, arthritis, rheumatism and period pain could perhaps be explained by their keeping in check the enzymes which are responsible for breaking down the body's natural opiates, endorphins.

It has long been known that nature's essential oils modify the body's electromagnetic fields, and as we discover more about the body's electrical patterns this

9

becomes an especially interesting aspect of them. According to the latest research, the body is a composite picture of electrical patterns, with each organ and area having its own unique pattern which becomes disturbed when the body is ill. Some of the most interesting research yet to be carried out on essential oils must surely be in this area. Perhaps the oils are attracted to particular organs by their vibrational pattern? The dextrorotatory and laevorotatory characteristics of essential oils should also be re-examined in view of our latest information about the body's electromagnetic fields.

There is also the possibility that the essential oils are natural 'capacitors' – able to store energy and release it when required. They could be found to be biological semi-conductors – able to amplify energy . . . literally boosting the system back into operation. Because the oils appear to be little changed when they leave the body, it is possible to classify them as 'bio-catalysts'. These are substances which aid or speed up chemical reactions in the body while remaining unchanged themselves. They may, in fact, be 'super-bio-catalysts', because of their electrical properties amplifying the effect of the chemical process.

There are many different areas in which essential oils should be further studied. To date, most of the research on them has been funded by the perfume or flavours and fragrance industries, which have been more concerned to identify the volatile elements – that is, those particles which float in the air and identify the molecules as 'lavender', 'jasmine' or 'rose'. This is what sells the product. In other words, they are more interested in what the oils *smell* like than what they *are*.

The positive effect of essential oils on blood circulation is well known (and not only related to their use in conjunction with massage during therapy). Increased blood flow improves the supply of oxygen and nutrients to the tissues and allows the efficient disposal of carbon dioxide and other waste products produced by cell metabolism. The immune system is improved by the general increase in movement and blood viscosity is decreased. A good blood circulation is absolutely vital to good health as it affects the working of every organ of the body, including the brain. Oxygen also helps to produce ATP (adenosine triphosphate), the body's fuel, by allowing glucose to be broken down into acetyl group molecules. The molecules are then carried off to the mitochondrion, the little power stations in cells, where they're subjected to the Krebs cycle to become pure ATP. Essential oils contain glucosytes which synthesize in the human body into glucose – the raw material of ATP. This may partly explain why some essential oils are so energizing. Another important factor in the efficacy of essential oils is their ability to reduce stress and tension, well-known suppressors of oxygen supply.

However, as we have seen, nature's essential oils are composed of hundreds of compounds, and tiny quantities of trace compounds may be what makes them so very special. With these oils, as with the human body, one cannot detach all the components from each other because they react together as an integrated whole. In human beings there are many additional constituents to the 'flesh and blood' and bone and body fluid that together make us what we are – some known and some unknown. We are learning continuously of new, important elements that go to make us healthy and vibrant. It is vital trace elements, like potassium, magnesium, copper and zinc, amongst others, which maintain balance within the human organism, and only by understanding their individual roles and integrated working can we appreciate what a very sophisticated machine the human body truly is. Biochemical researchers must be encouraged to take seriously the challenge of identifying the trace compounds in nature's essential oils, because until such time as all the components have been identified we cannot fully answer the question 'What are essential oils?' Let's just hope it doesn't take a thousand years!

HARVESTING THE PRECIOUS CROP

When harvesting the raw materials from which essential oils are extracted, timing is everything. Right now, somewhere in the world, an alarm clock is ringing to get the workers into the fields before dawn to pick the blossoms when the essential oil is most concentrated in their petals. It could be in Madagascar where they harvest the blossoms of the ylang-ylang tree, or in the south of France where they grow jasmine. They work between 4.30 a.m. and 9.30 a.m. at the foot of the Balkan Mountains in Bulgaria where they pick the Damascene rose.Outside this time-span, the essential oil content of the petals can be reduced by as much as 50 per cent.

Although most sweet-smelling flowers must have their petals processed immediately after harvest, many essential-oil-producing flowering tops and leaves, such as lavender and chamomile, are dried and shipped to other countries for distillation. This is possible because although sugars and starches will return from the leaf to the main body of the plant before the autumnal shedding, essential oils remain in the leaf or flowering top once they have arrived there.

The essential oil moves around plants not only on a daily basis, but on a seasonal one, too. Palma rosa oil is made from a grass which must be harvested before its flowers appear, while clove oil is made from flower buds after they have been picked and dried; pepper oil is made from the unripe berries, while coriander is harvested when its fruit is fully ripe. The delicate, white jasmine flower is carefully picked before it is one day old, but the sandalwood tree must be thirty years old and thirty feet high before its essential oil is fully developed and the government inspectors of the Indian province of Mysore decree it ready for pulverization and distillation into sandalwood oil. Some oils are as old as history itself; others are quite new. But whatever the oil, it is made from a particular part of a specific species of the plant and grown in very select areas of the world where the growing conditions are just right. This is a world-wide trade with oils coming from diverse destinations – China, Brazil, Turkey, Saudi Arabia, Indonesia, the United States, France, Réunion, Australia, Russia, Egypt, Zanzibar, Israel, Thailand, Java, Guatamala, Somalia and Spain, to name but a few.

It takes eight million hand-picked jasmine blooms to make one kilogram of 'absolute' from which the oil is made. There are only thirty harvesting days in Bulgaria, where about five tonnes of blooms produce one kilogram of oil. One good worker can pick about fifty kilograms of petals a day, enough to yield just a few precious drops of oil. Skill is required to coax the essential oil from the particular part of the plant in which it resides. Fennel and aniseed store their essential oil in the intercellular spaces in their tissue, and when the cells move apart from each other, minuscule canals form, full of oil. Some species have particular oil cells or resin cells, like cassia and cinnamon. Oranges and lemons form oil reservoirs when the walls of secretory cells gradually disintegrate. Other plants, like rosemary and sage, have glandular hairs, glandular cells or glandular scales on their surfaces – single- or multi-cell pockets, full of oil.

When producers of essential oil have identified exactly where the oil is to be found, they decide on the extraction method. The most widely used is called *distillation* and involves putting the material (cedarwood chippings, or the flowers and leaves of lavender, for example) in a still and forcing steam in from below which permeates the material. The volatile elements in the material rise together with the steam, and after condensation, turn into liquid form. Now the water and essential oil must be separated – some essential oils are lighter than water and are siphoned off the top; some are heavier and are siphoned off the bottom of the water-oil mix. The earliest still that we know of was invented by Maria Prophetissima, known as Maria the Jewess, who worked in Italy during the third century. The 'bain-marie' is named after her.

The oils in citrus fruit peel are extracted by *expression*. Until about 1930 this was done by hand with natural sponges. People hand-squeezed the essential oil into the sponge until it was saturated, then the oil was squeezed out of the sponge. These days expression is done by finely tuned machines, which must ensure that the rind is not exposed to heat as this changes the chemical structure and odour of the essential oils.

Enfleurage is an old method rarely used today because it's so labour intensive and time consuming. Certain types of flowers are placed in rows on fat which has been wiped across both surfaces of a piece of glass set in a frame. The fat draws the essential oil from the flower, and after a couple of days the frames are turned upside down so the old blooms fall off the fat and new blooms are put in their place. This process can go on for a couple of months, new flowers replacing the old, until eventually the fat is completely saturated, given the name pomade, and washed out with alcohol which is then evaporated, leaving the 'absolute'. *Enfleurage* is the easiest method of extraction to experiment with – Leonardo da Vinci, for example, used almond oil to soak up orange blossoms while he worked on perfumes at the court of Ludovico il Moro in Milan. Perhaps he was inspired by the ancient Indian method of putting jasmine flowers amongst warm sesame seeds, to infuse them with jasmine's aroma before pressing.

More commonly used today is *extraction*, a complicated procedure involving heating the raw material in a solvent, filtering, agitating with alcohol, cooling, filtering again, and then removing the alcohol by evaporation.

Depending upon the rarity and extraction method for particular oils, some can be expensive. This would be worrying if it weren't also the case that one doesn't actually need a great deal of essential oil, because these are the most concentrated life-essences known.

As ever, the demand for essential oils is greater than the supply. Growers around the world now rely on weather reports beamed down from satellites to best

14

manage their precious crops. In America today pepper-mint and spearmint are distilled within the body of huge harvesters as they roll through the fields. If that sounds highly technological, consider the fact that scientists are hoping to be able to raise essential oil glands by tissue culture in test tubes! But even today new methods of extraction are being developed which could lead to more of the essential oil's components being identified, as well as to purer product.

THE SUBTLE SENSE OF SMELL

We all know that someone who can't see is called 'blind', and that people who can't hear are called 'deaf', but what is the word to describe people who can't smell? The answer is 'anosmic'. In America alone, two million people suffer from anosmia. Most people who can't taste have anosmia too, because taste is actually a matter of smell – put a laundry peg on your nose when you eat dinner tonight and you'll see what I mean. Indeed, when you say 'This tastes good', it would be more accurate to say 'This smells good', because your taste buds can only distinguish between salty, sweet, bitter, sour and *unami*, while smell is at least ten thousand times more sensitive. *Unami* is a category that has recently been added by Japanese researchers; it denotes a savoury flavour, rather like fish or meat stock or monosodium glutamate, which westerners have no one word for. It's your nose which distinguishes between chicken soup and dishwater – not your 'good taste'!

In *The Man Who Mistook His Wife For a Hat and Other Clinical Tales*, neurologist Oliver Sacks tells the story of Sam, a medical student who, after a vivid dream that he was a bloodhound, woke up with a heightened sense of smell. He discovered that each person he passed on the street had a 'smell face' that was far more vivid than their 'sight face'. The assault of odour impressions did rather exhaust Sam for the three weeks that this episode lasted, yet even twenty years later he still occasionally yearned for that super-awareness which, in medical terms, is called hyperosmia. This condition is not unusual in people suffering from certain neuroses and psychoses, and in people being treated with L-dopa, a synthetic neurotransmitter, for inflammation of the brain; also those with Tourette's syndrome and some stroke patients report the same effect.

Another olfactory experience has been termed 'phantosmia' – hallucinations involving smell. This occurs when someone thinks they smell something when nothing is present. Schizophrenics, for example, sometimes think their bodies smell foul when they don't. This is known as dysosmia.

In the animal kingdom smell plays a crucial role in reproduction. For example, the male silkworm can detect a female five miles away by her aroma! However, it's been found that the male silkworm's sensitivity is only eight times greater than a human being's ability to perceive musk, possibly the most powerful odour known to man. It's not unusual for a gardener to be able to distinguish between the aromas of fifteen or more roses, so perhaps it's not surprising that the average healthy person can distinguish between ten and forty thousand odours. A professional 'nose' in the perfume, wine or whisky business, however, could have been trained to distinguish between one hundred thousand subtle aromas. To most of us, most of the time, our sense of smell is invisible. Yet it is most definitely there. And it is linked to sexuality. The amygdala, which receives messages about odour, deep within the brain, is not only also concerned with the expression of emotion, but has a direct link with the release of the hormones which control sexual development and activity. A quarter of those who have lost their sense of smell experience loss of libido.

One of the interesting things about smell is that it involves olfactory cells which are technically brain cells. Just behind the bridge of your nose there's a small, spoon-like structure which extends out from and is actually a part of the brain. This extraordinary object is called the olfactory bulb and from it olfactory nerve cells reach down to the inside of your nose. When an aroma particle floats into your nostril it makes a direct connection with these nerves and sparks off an immediate reaction in the brain. Aroma molecules set into action the limbic system, which is a complex network of structures and nerves constituting a neuronal circuit on which we find our centre for emotion and a crucial 'bottleneck' for memory. In other words, aroma, emotion and memory are inextricably linked. But that's not all. Through the limbic system, the hypothalamus and pituitary glands are stimulated, causing reactions in the autonomic nervous system and the endocrine (hormone) system, thus exerting an influence on nerves, hormones, body temperature, insulin production, appetite, thirst, calorific levels, digestion, stress, repulsion, sexual arousal and sex. (Now you know why Aromantics are so interested in smell!) As if all this weren't enough, the limbic system also connects with the thalamus and neocortex, giving aromas the ability to affect conscious thought and reaction. To summarize, then, what you smell affects just about everything from your emotions, memories and hormone levels to a whole range of vital physical processes, plus it can affect whether you think straight and get going, too!

But who notices smell except when dinner is about to be served, something is burning or the baby needs changing? More people than you might think. Science has confirmed a phenomenon which women have known from experience – a group of women living or working together tend to synchronize their periods. Apparently this happens because of a signal in the odour of their perspiration. Clearly, we smell more than we think we do. The connection between smell and hormone production is again confirmed by experiments which show that women who regularly smell a man's perspiration have more regular periods and girls begin their menstruation earlier when regularly in the company of men. And the connection works in the reverse direction, too – women perceive aromas best when they're ovulating and least when they're menstruating. For example, it's been found that women are one thousand times more sensitive to exaltolide, a chemical similar to testosterone, just before ovulation than earlier in the menstrual cycle.

In a recent scientific paper, zoologist Dr Michael Stoddart of the University of Tasmania reported that 'human beings are the most highly scented of the great apes'. We have apocrine sebaceous glands at the base of the hair follicles, under the arms and especially around the genitals, which are activated when we are sexually aroused, frightened or excited. They produce a highly complex blend of components, including some known as pheromones – odorous substances which are detected by others and produce psychological or behavioural changes in them. The existence of our secreting glands suggests to Dr Stoddart that human beings have 'a well-developed scent communication system' . . . whether we're aware of it or not! Certainly, Napoleon was aware of it. He asked Josephine not to bathe for several days before he was due to return from one of his victorious trips abroad. This might have been because of the axilla, an organ about a centimetre in size which secretes an oily sweat from the underarms chemically similar to the human sex hormones oestrogen and testosterone.

Pheromones send subtle messages to others of the same species, and in the animal world their role is impressive, to say the least. According to E.O. Oliver of Harvard University, 'One milligram of the trail pheromone of the leaf-cutter ant is enough to lead a small column three times around the world.' The highly complex and concentrated aromas produced by nature are obviously more powerful than their minuscule molecular size might suggest!

The extraordinary power and individuality of aroma molecules extends to plant life, too. For example, each river has its own aroma 'fingerprint', produced by the particular soils on the river bed and the plants in the river and along its shore. It's this 'aroma-river-print' that a salmon recognizes out at sea and follows all the way home so that she can spawn in the river of her birth, after perhaps several years and thousands of miles at sea. It's absolutely staggering that a fish can remember and locate in the vastness of the ocean the exact molecules that imprinted on its aroma memory on its original swim downstream, so long before. And it is just as amazing that the aroma molecules produced by the soils and plants in the home-stream can still be distinguished from other 'aroma-river-prints' after being flushed into the enormity of water that is the ocean.

Animals rely on their sense of smell to find 'home', mark out territory, find food, give warnings and identify one another, while human beings have evolved thinking neocortex brain cells and designed maps, supermarkets and legal writs, and we identify each other by our names. Nevertheless, we still produce highly powerful, if subtle, odorous substances, and our sense of smell hasn't gone away. It seems that when we were more primitive organisms smell was our main self-protection mechanism, and as we evolved, the central, primary area of the brain dealing with this function was gradually covered with grey thinking matter. In 1986, Dr Michael Shipley, a neurobiologist at the University of Cincinnati, was asked in *National Geographic* whether evolution had diminished human beings' sense of smell. He said that although we don't appear to be very conscious of smells, a large proportion of man's brain is still concerned with smell, and aromas have a very privileged and intimate access to those parts of the brain where we really live.

If we no longer rely on smell, it's become a con-firming mechanism that can exert a unique and power-ful influence on just about every important aspect of our lives, including the subconscious. Subtle isn't the word. Gas chromatography is a process that can detect a thousandth of a millionth of a gram of aroma substance. The human nose and brain detect substances a hundred

19

times smaller than that. It used to be widely accepted that the odour of a particular substance was related to the shape of its molecules until more and more smell-shape data was collected, and now that theory is looking distinctly shaky. What we do know is that in each nostril there are five million receptor cells concentrated in a tiny area the size of a shirt-button on each side behind the bridge of the nose, under the brain. These receptor cells are cilia, thread-like structures, and lying on top of them is a film of mucus. Although these ten million cilia all look exactly the same, scientists now believe they're actually composed of different proteins. When we breathe in, aroma molecules – all unique – roll on to the mucous layer and then penetrate this to bind with the receptor cells. They stay in contact like this for a second, a minute or several minutes, disconnect and make their way back through the mucus. When we breathe out, they float away again.

The suggestion that each cilia has a different protein composition points to 'chemical attraction', which explains how a particular aroma molecule manages to identify the exact cilia it needs to make the connection so that our brain registers 'This is an apple', or 'This is a tennis ball'. However, there are many elements involved which may also prove to be important in explaining the mechanism, including the electrostatic charge of the molecule, the ratio of fat:water content of the cilia, and the vibrational pattern produced by the distinctive shape of each molecule.

It will take scientists some time yet to solve this, and it is certainly an enormous challenge, but in the meantime society is waking up to the profound importance of the sense of smell and beginning to put what we do know to good use. As a method of absorption into the body, 'sniffing' is now considered effective enough to be utilized for taking contraceptives, steroids and vitamins.

The connection between aroma and emotion is being exploited by the fragrance and flavours industry. The world's largest company in this area, International

Flavours and Fragrances, is researching fragrances to relax; to lower blood pressure; to fall asleep; to wake up; to stay alert while learning, working or driving; to aid confidence; and to cope with depression, anxiety and other moods – all in order to make you feel good as well as smell good. The fragrance and flavours industry puts the 'soft' smell in your fabric conditioner, the 'alpine flowers' in your shampoo and the 'lemon' in your washing-up liquid. But it hasn't been as interested in the complex structure of natural aroma molecules as in replicating their aroma cheaply. So that 'lemon' is likely to be citral or, alternatively, ethyl acetate. The 'lily of the valley' in your soap is more likely to be hydroxycitronellal; the 'geranium' in your bubble bath, diphenyl oxide. The big questions for the future are whether the research at the world's universities into the sedative and stimulant properties of natural essential oils will be used by the fragrance and flavours industry to back up their use of these natural substances in their new 'mood' products, or will the 'jasmine' product to help you concentrate while studying just smell like jasmine and actually be benzyl acetate?

Fortunately, Aromantics don't have to worry whether they're getting the real thing! In this book you will be taking advantage of thousands of years of hands-on research. And you can take comfort in the knowledge that you will only be exposing your body and mind to the harmless and harmonious properties of natural products rather than subjecting yourself to the unknown cumulative effects of chemicals which, although supposedly harmless in themselves, could be very harmful when in conjunction with each other.

Let us remember that our sense of smell was our first, primary defence mechanism. Our reaction to smell is quicker, at 0.5 seconds, than to pain (0.9) or auditory stimuli (0.15). Scientists don't believe that brain cells regenerate themselves, but olfactory brain cells do – clearly underlining their importance. The sense of smell can be trained. So let us foster our subtle sense of smell using nature's essential oils and become Aromantic!

HOW THE ESSENTIAL OILS WORK AS APHRODISIACS

We shall be looking at eight different ways in which nature's essential oils work on the human organism so that sexual vibrancy is increased. Breaking the subject down into distinct mechanisms is only a device to achieve understanding and clarity because, in reality, the body–mind works as an integrated unit. In the past, the distinction between body and mind has been overstated. Not all the oils are aphrodisiac, and this section relates only to those which are. A particular oil may work as an aphrodisiac by just one of the mechanisms outlined, or it may involve two or three or more. In fact, in most cases the essential oils in this book have a compound effect on the compound you – body–mind. In a very general sense, we could say that the essential oils create harmony within the body–mind and give a feeling of well-being and self-confidence. This isn't the zonked-out self-confidence of alcohol consumption, nor the false effect of chemical drugs, which can not only have bad side effects, but also cause addiction.

There are some very important differences between natural and chemical/petroleum substances in terms of the body's ability to absorb and assimilate them and, therefore, in their respective abilities to do the job. The sixty trillion or so cells in the human body are in the constant process of synthesizing large molecules of proteins and fat, and what's so remarkable about these on-going, complex reactions is that they all happen in a pH-neutral environment at a more or less constant temperature. Science cannot replicate in the laboratory this most fundamental process, despite having access to high-technology equipment and chemical tools.

Essential oils, on the other hand, are themselves a miracle of nature and are in complete harmony with mankind. Indeed, without plant life, from which essential oils are, of course, derived, animals and man would be without the energy on which their lives depend. We owe the very air we breathe and the food we eat to plants, so why should we not expect them to help us in that most crucial function of life – procreation, which is all about sex!

Emotion

Emotion is, of course, the driving force behind choosing a partner, and it plays a vitally important role in the satisfying expression of love. Our emotional state at any particular time can act as a powerful aphrodisiac or, conversely, as an anaphrodisiac.

It has been known for a very long time that essential oils can have a profound effect on human emotions. The ancient Egyptians burnt a different aromatic substance at morning, noon and night in thanks to the sun god Re, and the sunset formula was a complex mix of sixteen ingredients known as 'kyphi', so delightful that it was later adopted by the Greeks and Romans. Plutarch described it thus: '[it] lulled one to sleep, allayed anxieties and brightened dreams . . . [and was] made of those things that delight most in the night'. In 1875 W.S. Watson reported in *The Medical Press and Circular* that odours had been having an exhilarating effect on the mentally ill. These days the effects of odours on the emotions are easily measured by the changes in electrical charge on the skin. Laboratories today throughout the world routinely produce research confirming the impact of aroma on emotion. Professor Paolo Rovesti from Milan is just one professional who believes that aromatherapy can provide a solution to those characteristics of our age – anxiety and depression.

All over the world, doctors, nurses and aromatherapists use essential oils. They use them as medicines upon the human body, and as agents to modify mood and emotion.

But if essential oils calm down, they also uplift!

Indian yogis have taught for millennia that sweet-smelling aroma – in the form of oils, herbs or incense – should be used to stimulate creativity and raise the spiritual element. This is, indeed, why aroma is an integral part of religious rituals in many denominations all over the world. In the Indian ecstasy cults, which date back possibly 6000 years and are still practised by some today, 'perfumes' are used in the rituals. Men of the Kaula sects anoint their partner with oil of jasmine on the hands, patchouli on the cheeks and breasts, spikenard for the hair, musk for the mons Veneris, sandalwood on the thighs and saffron on the feet. Sexual yoga teaches that the sense of smell is associated with the primary 'prana', the upward-moving vitality.

On a more mundane level, many clinical–psychological tests have proved that 'feeling better' is a major factor in getting better. But why wait until we're ill? Emotional problems tend to drag us into a negative vortex so we can't handle even the simplest of daily tasks without agitation and irritability. Depression can easily set in if we allow things to get on top of us. But the human condition is all about ups and downs. We're all prone to emotional troubles every now and again, and what better to balance us out than nature's relaxing and uplifting little helpmates?

Conscious Thought and Reaction

It is now an established scientific fact that aroma affects a person's ability to think more clearly and perform tasks more efficiently. The Tokyo construction company, Shimizu, use lemon fragrance in their self-devised, central air-circulating system to increase productivity in their keypunch operators. They must think it worth it at around $20,000 a room. Shimizu now have a subsidiary marketing the system in America. Not that America is new to aroma generation. You can buy your very own desktop aroma unit for $100.

In *Fragrant Sensuality* you will find essential oils and

formulas to help conscious thought and reaction, because being able to deal effectively with the intellectual pressures of modern life has great bearing on a person's sexual interest and response. Being in control of the work-world situation directly influences levels of self-confidence which, in turn, affect sex. As a self-aphrodisiac, there's none better than the knowledge that we can handle whatever life throws at us, and as an aphrodisiac for the opposite sex, self-confidence is as nectar to the bee!

Pressure at work affects us all, and on the computerized factory assembly line, not being on the ball can lose you more than your job. The stress and tension it causes are major pleasure suppressors, and just as real for women if, in the bedroom, more noticeable for men. Everything in life is interrelated: work and play, day and night. All too often people turn to stimulants which cloud the mind or pull them into a negative, unhelpful vortex. Essential oils, on the other hand, give you a very real mental liberation, not an escape. Your mental faculties will be increased, not impaired or imprisoned. Essential oils leave you strong, not weak; aware, not half-blitzed; on your feet, not legless.

And when you're better able to cope with the ever-present hurly-burly of professional life, you can better enjoy that most natural activity – making love. Essential oils, moreover, provide the mind with an extraordinary clarity that can perhaps best be described as super-perception. The Aromantic mind can see how good life and love can be.

The Nervous System

In 1980, researchers at Hammersmith Hospital in London revealed a new branch of the autonomic system – which they have called the 'peptidergic' – and reminded us all that human physiology is not yet entirely mapped. However, I don't want to go into the whole subject of the human nervous system here, but to concentrate on one aspect of it – the delicate balance between the sympathetic and parasympathetic.

These two are, in effect, a pair of 'on' and 'off' switches, using chemicals as the force to effect changes in the working of those organs under their control. For example, the parasympathetic nerves slow the beat of the heart, while the activity of the sympathetic increases the beat. The sympathetic branch uses adrenaline (as well as noradrenaline and other substances), which is fairly well known as the 'fright, flight, fight' hormone which comes to our aid in emergencies. It's also this sympathetic/adrenaline system which causes ejaculation. Premature ejaculation occurs when a man can't control the amount of adrenaline that his brain is directing to be released into the bloodstream – a result of over-excitement, fear or anxiety.

Premature ejaculation, impotence, non-orgasm in women, and low levels of arousal are all due to a degree of imbalance between the two halves: the parasympathetic which prepares for orgasm and the sympathetic which achieves it. Men tend to have an overactive sympathetic – premature ejaculation, and women an underactive one – non-orgasm. This is very much a simplification of the whole process involved, but you can see how important the nervous system is to us. So it has ever been. In ancient Indian parlance, men were compared to fire (quick to ignite and easily extinguished) while women were compared to water (slow to come to the boil, but once there, the temperature can easily be maintained).

The early research into the autonomic nervous system was carried out on men returning from war and on women who had been raped, who, because of an overdose of the 'fright' hormone, adrenaline, had experienced serious changes in their brain biochemistry. This teaches us still today that although a cause might be emotional, its effect will be chemical.

However, there are no emotional virgins, and the sexuality of everyone, therefore, is prone to disturbance. Often a vicious cycle develops so that, for example, Jack feels under pressure to perform, the anxiety causes the adrenaline to flow, which triggers ejaculation, ruining his 'performance' and thus compounding his problem.

The nervous system works as an integrated unit – and balance is everything! Essential oils get straight to the nervous system, and have for millennia been used as balancers of the two halves of the autonomic nervous system.

A number of oils have been tested for their influence on the sympathetic branch of the nervous system by Professor Shizuo Torii of Toho University in Japan, and his findings confirm our empirical knowledge. He found that the action of the sympathetic nervous system was increased by jasmine, ylang-ylang, peppermint, rose, patchouli, neroli, clove, bois de rose and basil; while its activity was decreased by marjoram, sandalwood, lemon, chamomile and bergamot.

The knowledgeable use of nature's oils can exert an influence over the on-off mechanism of the nervous system, thus affecting sexuality. But let us not forget that balance and control in sexuality is not just about being able to avert disaster, but about building up new highs!

Hormones

Psychopharmacologists are awash with enkephalins, dynorphin, endorphins and beta-endorphins, like dopamine, acetylecholine, and casomorphin, not to mention phenylethylamine. And they're linking them with our pleasure receptors in the brain. We are obviously designed to have fun.

It's not only scientists that are interested in fun. It will come as no surprise to Aromantics that MDMA (also known as 'ecstasy') was originally synthesized from a chemical in nutmeg. Nobody has yet proved that similarly interesting chemicals do not exist in other natural products, such as jasmine and rose, which

27

human beings have been using to provide pleasure for millennia.

So far, over fifty hormones have been identified in the human body – not all of them, of course, related to sex. Hormones are chemical messengers which are secreted into the bloodstream by endocrine glands or produced during nerve impulse transmission. Some of the glands are quite specifically hormonal in their activity, like the pituitary which produces no less than eight hormones, or the adrenal glands, while others are more commonly thought of as organs, like the pancreas. Even the heart secretes its own hormone which, it is thought, could be a factor in regulating blood pressure.

With all hormonal activity, again, balance is everything. For example, inhibin and stimulin are a pair of on-off switches that between them effect the production of sperm and the release of ova. A single physical process can involve a long chain of many hormones, and synchronization between all the hormonal activity is vital to good health.

In the essential oils we seem to have nature's very own hormone replacement therapy. Geranium and eucalyptus are used in medicinal aromatherapy in the treatment of diabetes, the condition caused by a deficiency of the hormone insulin. Female reproductive problems can be treated with clary-sage, fennel and the rose family of essential oils. Research reveals that certain oils are very similar to certain hormones, for example oestrogen and progesterone. Perner and Zenife have proved the effects of particular oils on the menstrual cycle, which is, of course, a hormonal activity.

Not all essential oils can be called a part of nature's hormone replacement therapy. Only certain oils have been observed in research or therapeutic practice to have these effects; but many are relaxants, and relaxation not only helps hormone release and balance and improves the body's defence mechanisms, but is also an important element in being able to enjoy sexuality to the full.

As an aphrodisiac, then, nature's essential oils relax; some specifically work on the sexual hormones, stimulating sexual activity; and generally they help us to feel well and look good. And a healthy, happy person has always been a powerful aphrodisiac to the opposite sex.

Silent Biological Messengers

Plants, insects, animals and human beings have silent biological messengers. The messages are to do with life and death – sexual attraction, reproduction and defence against attack. In 1982, American biologists Drs Orians and Rhoades first discovered that trees send each other 'air mail' aroma messages, warning of attack by insects. Flowers and plants send insects and animals aroma messages saying, 'Come here' or 'Go away', depending on the species and whether the plant has a symbiotic relationship with it.

Human beings react strongly to the sexual glandular secretions of certain animals – the civet cat, the castor-yielding beaver, and most especially the musk deer. Indeed, perfumers will pay huge sums of money to obtain these substances so they can be included in their products. Certain essential oils, such as ambrette and angelica, mimic the aroma of musk.

But we don't need musk. Human beings send each other messages in the form of pheromones. In studies it's been shown that men find women's odour most alluring during ovulation. We also know that men respond to this odour by producing their own which, in turn has an aphrodisiac effect on the woman. Emily Jacobs, working at St Thomas's Hospital in London, found that vaginal secretions daubed on the woman's chest encouraged lovemaking. You can see why the word 'pheromone' was taken from the two Greek words, *pherein* – to bear along – and *hormon* – an excitement! The silent biological messengers affect not only the consummation of sex but the development of it. Men kept in olfactory isolation from females during puberty produce less facial hair; conversely, men who have been exposed to the female smell and/or essential oils can often grow hair where none grew before!

If hormones are the body's internal message system, pheromones send messages out. Research psychologist Michael J. Russell from the University of California Medical Center suggests that before lovemaking commences, the apocrine glands all over the body, but especially in the face, release odiferous signals. This is part of the reason there is such pleasure in kissing. The whole subject of human pheromone production is one of much scientific debate. However, anyone who has seen Lennart Nilsson's magnificent photographs of pheromones magnified 400,000 times must surely be impressed.

Certainly in the animal kingdom, pheromones are crucial. The sexual cycle of the female sheep, goat and certain monkeys is governed by the release of pheromones in the male. It is the pheromones released when a female dog is in heat that brings the dogs on the other side of the park running. Conversely, if you plug the nose of a male rhesus monkey, it will appear to defy nature and ignore the females in heat. The recipient of the male hamster's sexual attention needn't be a hamster because researchers have shown that the scent from a female hamster's vagina, if smeared on balls of string, torches and rubber toys, will elicit the same response.

Human beings are more highly evolved, of course, and our responses are, fortunately, more subtle. Unless we're under hypnosis, the pre-frontal lobe, which is absent in animals, filters instinct. We behave ourselves even if we don't want to.

Some flowers mimic the pheromones of insects, thus achieving their own pollination. The powerfully scented white flowers attract the moth, their perfume exuding most before the day begins, when the moths are about. How a flower manages to replicate an insect's silent biological messenger is a question we cannot answer, but clearly flowers are 'smart'. Smart people too, have for millennia been using essential oils for the purpose of attraction and propagation: in other words, for making love.

Perfumery is an old, complex and subtle science, and because each person's aroma preference is so unique, it may take you a little time to identify the Aromantic essential oils that your partner finds particularly exciting. But think what fun you'll have in the trying!

Health and Beauty

It is in the area of health and beauty, rather than sex, that the use of nature's essential oils is best known. If you're feeling good, self-confidence is running high, and the fact that you're looking good no doubt helps too! Ill health, pain or discomfort deplete energy which could be better spent on more positive things – like making love. In this book I have given you some formulas to deal with physical problems that directly affect sexuality, from infections to muscle fatigue. If you are already well, the essential oils tone the physical system and elevate your mood. In this process, the sexual organs are relaxed, toned and invigorated, too.

The natural essential oils work on the physical body in many diverse ways, but in a general sense they're excellent for all-round physical vigour because, as Dr Jean Valnet points out, one of their abilities is to increase blood supply to the tissues which assists both the cell regeneration and the 'detergent action' of the white blood corpuscles. They are carried throughout the whole body, leading to an internal and external revitalization and radiance.

Aesthetic Considerations

Perfumes are an aesthetic delight, but they're not entirely innocent. A famous French perfumer, Pierre Blaizot, once admitted that fragrances in a perfume laboratory are so erotic that a man with normal sexual desires is in danger of being driven to distraction and, indeed, relapses in virtue. Poor M. Blaizot and his associates have suffered so that you and I can drive our partner to 'distraction' too! For perfumes undoubtedly attract. We want to be closer to the delicious smell, to savour the experience. And we all know that there is no greater aphrodisiac than the idea that someone finds us attractive, even if it's initially our perfume that they are trying to get close to. Wearing a delightful aroma can even make passers-by stop in their tracks to identify where the aroma is coming from. The mundane world stops; romance enters in.

From the consumer's point of view, aesthetic considerations are to do with becoming oneself, expressing one's personality through aroma. Perfume confirms our individuality to others and to ourselves. It 'fixes' us in one spot for a moment in time. This process is very subtle, so that an aroma worn to go to the office won't seem appropriate at the gym, nor on a hot date with the lover. We wear perfumes like clothes from the wardrobe. At least, women do. With Aromantics, however, men can benefit, too, from the 'filling out' mechanism, with the subtle aromas and methods of use made possible with nature's essential oils. He can begin his day with an invigorating grapefruit shower; have a sniff of basil, just before going in to the crucial business meeting, from the bottle he keeps in his desk drawer; and have a clary-sage bath before he goes out for a euphoric evening!

The subtlety of the character-filling-out mechanism means that one can really *be* the person one would like to be at any particular time – and it won't just be an auto-suggestory illusion. Moreover, with essential oils one can make formulas very easily, so that with just a few basic ingredients one can produce a huge variety of aroma/emotion effects by changing the ratios of each oil that's included. In this way, an Aromantic can explore the deep, mercurial aspects of their character, so that at any time one can feel and say with confidence, 'This is me' and, moreover, like it! The essential oils, then, work as an aphrodisiac in this respect because a person who is truly themselves, and happy, is powerfully attractive to the opposite sex.

Memory

Researchers have found that if we soon forget things we see and hear, odours we remember for a lifetime. Indeed, so powerful is the odour–memory connection that students are being advised to study with an aroma present. It doesn't matter which aroma is used – good or bad – so long as it's near again during exams, when all those facts come flooding back.

We all have a unique reaction to particular smells because we've all had a personal history of exposure to aromas with their associated emotional connections. A particular oil has its own properties, but your memory can override all that if the aroma has a strong emotional connotation for you. An awareness of this process means that we can 'cash in' on the good aroma-memory-emotion connections or 'reprogramme' the ones that are doing us no good. This is a subject that deserves more space and, indeed, the next section is devoted to it. But as a quick example, suppose your most exciting sexual experience happened when you were eighteen, behind a trellis of jasmine in the garden on a warm summer night. Any time in the future when you smell jasmine again, this sexy memory floods back. If you are aware of the connection, you can make the memory work for you by using jasmine. Napoleon's mistress, Josephine, obviously knew of this effect when, spurned by her lover in favour of Marie-Louise, she drenched the palace bedrooms with musk, her own favourite perfume and notoriously retentive. Indeed, the musk could still be smelt long after all concerned had moved on. How Napoleon reacted to the musk we simply do not know, but it sent Marie-Louise into a scurry as she rushed through the palace, saturating it in the perfume Napoleon would associate with her – violets.

Memory can work as an anaphrodisiac as well. A particular aroma can turn you off the idea of making love, and you may not realize why. Emotional ghosts can, however, be cleared out of the memory cupboard with Aromantic awareness. But that's another subject . . .

Aromantic Awareness

Choosing aromas is very much a matter of personal taste. No single perfume will appeal to everyone; indeed, it can both delight and repel. This is one reason why *Fragrant Sensuality* offers you choices.

Aroma preference is a matter of learning. When you were born you had a blank 'odour-sheet', and you slowly started to associate specific aromas with particular emotions you experienced at the time you smelt the aroma. The linking of aroma with emotion and long- and short-term memory is a vital self-protection mechanism. We learn to beware of things that are dangerous (like burning furniture) and recognize things that are good for us (like mother), and we recognize these things through smell with the help of memory. Dr Betelheim, an American psychoanalyst working with toddlers, has found that those left with an item of mother's clothing were content to be left.

Scientists claim that an infant can recognize the odour of its mother's milk by the time it is between six and fourteen days old. The first important odour goes down on the odour-sheet with the connection, 'This is good, it satisfies my hunger and makes me feel secure'. Let's say this baby's loving father happened to smoke a pipe. A second entry in the memory-bank would be 'Pipe smoke reminds me of happy times, sitting on my father's lap'. A baby thus collects good associations and emotions. Now let's suppose that this baby was looked after by a cruel nursemaid who slapped the baby when it cried (and the parents weren't looking), and that the nurse wore lavender-based perfume. The aroma of lavender goes down with the connection, 'I smell lavender, I feel uncomfortable and nervous'. This process goes on year after year, all completely subconsciously perhaps, until the child becomes a man or woman and the blank odour-sheet becomes a complex 'computer program' of aroma.

We all have a subconscious memory-bank which is loaded with good and bad associations. When we smell a long-forgotten aroma, the memory of a particular person, event or whole period of life floods back to us, complete with emotional associations. A grown man smells lavender and a shiver runs down his back . . . and he may not even know why. When we understand the role aroma can play in directing our moods and emotions we can make good use of it to enhance our lives. This is because the computer program is always being added to, not only in the usual subconscious way, but it can be consciously added to, too. We will all make aroma–memory–emotion associations until the day we die.

Aroma programming happens to us all. Suppose you were wearing patchouli when your partner came home in a filthy mood and you had a blazing row. Without even realizing it, his or her memory-bank has registered patchouli = partner = bad experience. Whatever you do, don't carry over this association into the bedroom. Have a shower or bath, put another aroma on yourself, and in this way you're consciously making sure that at least one part of the association (patchouli = bad experience) has been washed away. Choose an aroma to wear at this time which has good associations for your partner, or one that has as yet no associations.

Sometimes we may need aroma 'reprogramming'. For example, if you don't like the aroma of oranges this could be because of an emotion–memory imprint established with an unpleasant childhood experience. Perhaps you stole an orange from the cupboard and got caught as you were eating it – smell and taste are linked – you got spanked and sent to bed without any supper. Perhaps as you were lying there crying and feeling sorry for yourself, you heard your parents arguing over the incident and with this sound ringing in your ears, you finally fell asleep . . . the tears still wet on your little face. The next morning you might have forgotten the whole ghastly affair, but your subconscious did not. End result: whenever you smell oranges you feel flooded with an odd, inexplicable feeling of guilt, pain, hunger, self-pity and fear. But there really is no value in having useless, negative subconscious associations. In this instance, you're just depriving yourself of oranges and vitamin C. What you need now is to put the aroma in a new, positive context. Choose a relaxing day and surround yourself with as many good elements as you can. Put your favourite music on the tape deck. Ask your partner, or a genuine friend, to be present to help you out. Now, put a couple of drops of orange oil on a source of heat in the room and breathe deeply, with eyes closed and thinking only of the things in life you most like. If you're with someone, ask them to gently caress your hair, back or whatever, as if you were a cat just enjoying the warmth of a loving, human touch. Indulge yourself in whatever pleasure you can think of to build up a new program for the aroma of orange so that when you next smell it, it won't immediately evoke uncomfortable feelings, but feelings of security, love and happiness.

Don't worry that there's a danger of associating punishment with pleasure and developing a confused attitude. You will retain the two experiences as separate entries on your limbic system, but the new, pleasurable experience and sensation will overlay the old, unpleasant one. Some old memories are more powerful than others and you may need to overlay the bad experience with good more than once, but eventually the unpleasant association will retreat.

Clearing the emotional ghosts out of the cupboard by deliberately using aroma could be very important for the many people who find themselves unaccountably upset on a regular basis and can't understand why. With odour-awareness, we can take more control of our lives. Suppose another little boy used to be beaten by his father with a leather strap and now he finds himself working as a lawyer in an office that is furnished with big leather sofas. He may not immediately be able to understand why he 'just feels uncomfortable' working in this firm, but with odour-awareness he can apply his mind to search for the negative connection and take steps to overcome the problem. In this case, he should take an aroma, sandalwood, for example, and use it only for especially wonderful moments – making love, listening to his favourite music or whatever. Then, when he goes to the office, he can put 2-3 drops of sandalwood oil on to a heat source so that it permeates his working environment. In this way, he's overlaying the original, negative aroma connection with a new, positive one.

It's important to realize the impact one's mother's perfume or father's aftershave can have on later life. Lovers should be aware of avoiding the aroma each other's parents used. If your father gives a bottle of his favourite aftershave to your lover it shouldn't even be taken out of the box! You'd find it difficult to experience your lover as a sexual partner when his aroma just reminds you of your father. Instead, there would be an inexplicable discomfort. By the same token, if your lover buys you a perfume because it was the one his mother wore, pretend to lose it! I mean, are you sure you want him to be flooded with memories of his mother when you are both lying there in bed?

So far, we've discussed Aromantic awareness in terms of the past. But what about the future? Well, here too Aromantic awareness can be put to good use. To start with, it can get you the job! Industrial psychologist Dr Robert Barron, and his team at Purdue University, USA, were surprised by the results of their research into the effects of wearing perfume or aftershave at job interviews. Male interviewers tended to react nega- tively to male applicants wearing aftershave and female applicants wearing perfume and gave them lower evaluations, despite the fact that their qualifications matched other, non-perfumed applicants. Women interviewers, on the other hand, had a neutral or favourable reaction to perfumed contestants.

It seems that male interviewers have difficulty in filtering out personal, grooming characteristics from purely professional ones; while women interviewers, if their reaction was favourable rather than neutral, saw perfumes as good grooming. Clearly, it's worth finding out if your interviewer is male or female, but as the interviewer might change due to unforeseen circumstances at the last minute, it may be altogether safer to go Aromantic! You could start your day by having a shower or bath with one of the subtle essential oils – a 'Confidence booster' – on page 121 perhaps, or one of the 'Go for it!' formulas on page 122.

You've probably all experienced how a particular perfume or aftershave reminds you of a particular person, and especially a person with whom you had a close, emotional relationship. Years after you broke up, all you have to do is smell that aroma again and you remember that person in an emotional sense, even if you can no longer recall the exact shape of their face. It's this aspect of aroma's remarkable power that can be put to good use to ensure that you make a lasting impression (and I mean lasting) on your lover of today.

Buy a perfume or aftershave that's just been put on the market, preferably one produced by a famous perfume house, because that has a stronger likelihood of remaining on the market for years to come. Use this perfume or aftershave on yourself lavishly for at least a week, or on nine consecutive dates if you're not living together and, whenever you see your lover during this period, make an extra special effort to be loving, caring, sharing, supportive and sexy – all those positive things that go to make a good relationship. Avoid arguments at all costs. And be absolutely sure that your partner actually likes the aroma of the perfume or aftershave. The sexier things are now between you, the better.

This aroma will now be imprinted on your lover's limbic brain so that years later, even when they're eighty years old, whenever they smell that aroma, it will remind them of you. In the years to come your present passion may not remember your name or face, but the sensation of you will, with the perfume, last for ever. When they're living in the old people's home and the new nurse comes on duty wearing the 'classic' aroma, your lover will wistfully remember their passionate youth (and, would they but know it, that memory will be of you). This is the Aromantic meaning of 'spreading a little happiness'!

I have a friend who has always used this 'memory imprint' method and she receives phone calls from ex-lovers like nobody else I know. Some phone saying 'I just thought I'd call to see how you're doing', and others know why they call: 'I smelt your perfume today and it reminded me of our good times together so I thought I'd call . . . how are you?'

Good memories should be what love is all about . . . but make sure *you're* the one your lover remembers! If your lover brings you a perfume they say they smelt before and liked, beware, you may be wearing an aroma that provides your partner (subconsciously perhaps) with a reminder of a former lover. If that's the case, you'd better get going and make Aromantic awareness work for *you*!

DISCOVERING THE AROMANTIC YOU

When we talk Aromantics, we're not only talking sweet smells, but also emotions, moods, memories, mental stimulation, physical health and a confident glow. Aromantics is about all-round fulfilment.

Looking through humanity's aroma-past, we see that every nation or religious group inextricably linked sweet smells with spirituality. The Latin *per fumin* – through smoke – is about incense burning and rising to greet the gods. People realized that aroma is one of the

Earth's most valuable and delightful products – a bonus that keeps body and soul together. After all, there's no reason why the deity needed to make some of the world's natural products so fabulous a delight to the senses. Plant pheromones could be like animal pheromones – rather unpleasant to smell. But they're not. Our ancestors marvelled at this fact, taking it as a sign of the deity's love of us. We know that the aroma also serves as a warning pesticide and is the plant's natural antibacterial agent which we, too, can benefit from. Indeed, its sweet aroma draws us to it, almost as if by design, to partake of the aromas or ingest the leaves in our culinary habits. Our scientific knowledge should make us even more in awe of the beauty of creation than our ancestors were, as we realize its aromatic design.

From what we now know about the psychological effects of odour, it would be unrealistic to hold the bland, old-fashioned view that people in times past merely used aroma to cover up bad smells. It is far more likely that they realized the uplifting mental and emotional properties of aroma, just as we do. Or why else would the classical poets discuss the finer points of metaphysics while having their feet rubbed with aromatic oils? And it's interesting to note that the Greek ladies rubbed marjoram oil on their heads – was that the Valium of the classical age?

In what is thought to be the first novel ever written, the *Tale of Genji*, the author, Lady Murasaki, describes 'incense parties' that took place in the tenth-century Japanese palaces. Apparently, the players 'listened' to various aromas, and from them imagined ever-more elaborate stories. In the museums and antique shops of Japan you can see many beautiful examples of the incense-game boxes used to store the various aromatics which participants had to guess. Today the Japanese play *Kodo*, a commercially packaged game whereby scented wooden sticks are put in warm ashes to release the aroma, which has to be guessed by the players. But aroma, for the Japanese, has not simply been about having fun. In the seventeenth and eighteenth centuries there were entire schools of aroma, the *Shino-ryu*, founded by the Samurai, and the *Oiye-ryu*, organized by the courtiers of the imperial palace, teaching how incense should be used both personally and in groups, to develop discipline and honour.

All the most interesting characters of history used perfumes – which were then, of course, nature's essential oils, rather than the chemical copies we know today. Cleopatra made sure of her supply by having an enormously extravagant garden which was tended by her very own perfumers. We know from the records kept by his perfumer, Chardin, that Napoleon's consumption of rosemary eau de cologne was prodigious – 162 bottles in the first three months of 1806 alone. What we don't know is whether Napoleon chose rosemary for its vitality-restoring properties as he liberally splashed it on himself after his bath, as has been reported, or whether he appreciated more its highly antiseptic quality on the battlefield, or its brain-stimulating properties as he planned his army's manoeuvres in the next attack. Perhaps it was the combination of properties that made him such a fan. For his empress, Josephine, Napoleon bought the best Spanish jasmine, and sent her perfumes from his 'trips' abroad.

In *Fragrant Sensuality* some of the secrets of aroma will be revealed to you. As aroma works on the physical, emotional and spiritual at the same time, with clever blending everything is possible. You can learn to balance out you and your lover's characteristics. You can heal yourself while smelling good at the same time. You can be fortified and handle the day-to-day routine with confidence. In 'Aromantic woman' and 'Aromantic man' we shall look at the oils and formulas which will bring you sexual well-being and help you realize your true sexual potential.

Fragrant Sensuality is a journey of adventure in nature's garden of delights and it is there you will discover the Aromantic you!

2

How To Use Nature's Essential Oils

THINGS YOU SHOULD KNOW ABOUT USING ESSENTIAL OILS

Like human beings, essential oils have complex characters. Just as a person can perform many varied tasks and roles, so too can the oils. A man can be flexible so that he's a miner, a computer whizz, a singer, a footballer, a husband, and a father and member of the St John Ambulance Brigade, depending on the time of week and the role required of him. Likewise, each oil is capable of many different roles, and they aren't mutually exclusive, so you will see an oil being used for many different purposes. This isn't a contradiction, but a reflection of the deep richness and beauty of nature.

When you put two people together, you make a unique relationship. When you put two or more oils together, you make a totally new organic compound. It's important to recognize this fact, because you may see a formula in a particular section of this book containing an oil which isn't listed in this chapter, or in 'Aromantic woman' or 'Aromantic man'. This isn't an omission: I used that oil in the formula and made a completely new compound, quite different from the original single oil. Oils cannot be taken out of the context of the formulas in which they occur. Just follow the directions!

With essential oils, more is not always best. Indeed, in some cases results are more effective when the oil has been diluted in greater volumes of base-oil or water. By the same token, when I offer you a choice of formulas for a particular situation and there are twenty-four drops in one, thirty in another, and twenty-eight in the third, don't think that the formula with thirty drops is stronger and more effective. The number of drops isn't as important as the potency of an individual oil and, more than this, the potency of the oils when in combination with each other.

Never think that using neat essential oil will speed up the process of healing. These are extremely concentrated substances and they need to be diluted. Using them neat is as pointless as drinking cordial neat.

Generally speaking, you'll find that the essential oils have a cumulative effect. You might find that your chosen essential oil or formula meets your need so fast you forget you ever had a need! On the other hand you might need to use the oil or formula for a week or so. It all depends on the depth and nature of the need. So be patient, give the oil or formula a chance to work, and if it isn't working, simply switch to an alternative oil or formula – and alternatives are always provided.

Some methods of use are more effective than others. Generally speaking, massage oil is the most effective because it combines absorption into the body via the skin with the direct brain connection through inhalation when you're applying the oil to your body. Direct inhalation is also very effective – simply sniffing the oil from the bottle or putting it on to a tissue and sniffing that. Baths are effective because the oil is absorbed through both the body and the nose. Room diffusers or the other room methods (candles, room sprays, water bowls, humidifiers and heat-sources) are less direct and more subtle. They are the gentle way.

Watch out for the directions involving spoonfuls of base-oil in which to dilute the essential oil. Sometimes I say teaspoon, and sometimes it's dessertspoon or tablespoon – so read the instructions carefully.

You will need some clean, dry bottles to make your formulas in. These should be brown or dark-coloured glass so the light doesn't affect the essential oils. Ask your pharmacist to sell you some in the sizes you require – the size will probably be imprinted on the bottom of the bottle. If it doesn't incorporate a dropper ask your pharmacist to sell you one separately, so you can ensure correct measurement. Store the bottles away from heat, light and damp.

For some of the treatments, especially the douches in 'Aromantic woman', I have specified 'pure' water. This means either bottled spring water or boiled tap water which has been allowed to cool to body temperature.

PURITY

If you were to attend an auction of essential oils, you'd see very clearly that different oils have very different prices. On my current wholesale list jasmine is ninety-two times the price of grapefruit and, less dramatically, sandalwood is four times the cost of lime. Prices vary so tremendously because each crop is subject to different conditions – the cost of harvesting and processing, the distance it has to travel to reach the auction, the supply and demand factor, and like any crop, the particular weather and growing conditions of the season. The best suppliers to the public sell their ranges of essential oils in a way that accurately reflects the vastly different conditions that each oil is subject to.

You need to discriminate when choosing your supplier. When someone adulterates the essential oil and puts a label on it saying 'Pure essential oil', they're not breaking the law, because it is essential oil – but it might not be the particular oil you think you're buying. You can yourself make a very plausible imitation aroma of the expensive carnation oil by combining ylang-ylang and black pepper, both of which are much cheaper. But you obviously won't have pure carnation oil, and although it might smell like carnation, it won't have the molecular structure or be capable of carrying out carnation's jobs.

Some suppliers sell products which cannot be called 'pure essential oil' because they are diluted into base-oils like almond, apricot, peach, grapeseed, hazelnut, soya, etc. These diluted products are easier to distinguish from the real thing because they'll be oily. Nature's essential 'oils' are not, in fact, oily – the term 'oil' is something of a misnomer. You can see the difference between essential oils and other vegetable or petroleum-based oils by comparing their drops on a piece of blotting paper – all other oils sit there in an oily patch, while the essential oils impregnate the paper, then evaporate and disperse, leaving no oily patch. If your 'essential oil' leaves an oily patch, the product could be suspect. Bear in mind, however, that there is enormous variation in the pure product – vetiver is dark-coloured and viscous, while lavender is more like water.

So, that was the bad news, here's the good: because essential oils can so easily be adulterated with cheaper essential oils, or diluted with base-oils, there's usually no need for the naughty supplier to add chemicals. That's something!

Price comparison is a good guide – if you can buy rose Bulgar at the same price as lavender, something is wrong . . . with the rose Bulgar. Comparison between suppliers is your best guide, so shop around, and if in doubt go for the most expensive. (We use such small quantities of the real thing that they still won't be too expensive, so don't worry.) If you find two ranges that are the same price and you aren't sure which is the best, again, don't worry too much. The essential oils are like love – you'll know the real thing when it comes along. You can find the address of one reputable mail-order supplier at the end of this book.

Be prepared for changes in price. There are vintage years in the growing of the oil-producing plants, just as there are vintage years in the growing of wine-grapes. Nature is unpredictable, and this is precisely why the chemical-based aroma industry can't be expected to enthusiastically forgo its easily managed factories for vast fields of flowers. Instead, it tries to replicate the effects produced by nature's essential oils, aware perhaps more than any of us that the miracles of science cannot yet match the miracles of nature.

But, ultimately, the quality of any product depends on the demands of the consumer – you. If we all demand the highest standards of purity, we can, together, make sure that we receive them.

SYNERGISTIC BLENDS AND MAKING YOUR OWN FORMULAS

In the hands of an artist the essential oils can be made to produce a masterpiece. The artistry comes from knowing which combinations mix well together, and the masterpiece is produced when harmony is accomplished by the total work.

One could compare the whole process to painting a picture. Both sets of raw materials are beautiful – what could be more delightful than the golden yellow of daffodils or the clear blue of a summer's sky? And all of nature's essential oils are, in themselves, beautiful too. The artist can mix the yellow and blue together to make green – and a whole range of greens, depending on the ratio of yellow to blue. And you can mix two essential oils together to make a completely new organic compound – and many different compounds, depending on the ratios you use. The artist can produce an enormous variety of colours from the three primary colours – yellow, red and blue – and you and I can produce an infinite number of blends from the vast number of essential oils.

Synergistic blends are combinations of essential oils which create unique energy and vibrational patterns.

The advantage in making a synergistic blend is that one can include a number of oils that if used in a straight formula would be one half, one quarter, or even less, of one drop (which would, of course, be difficult to measure out). By mixing a synergistic blend we can provide all the correct oils and in the correct proportions – albeit minuscule ones. The combinations allowed by synergistic blends make up totally new compounds (as do straight formulas, of course) which are very subtle and despite their sometimes small components, very powerful: they are more than the sum of their parts.

My synergistic blends are harmonious wholes, blended after many years of experience in using the tools of my trade. Specialist therapists design individual formulas for their patients and these formulas can vary on each visit, because people change with time and have new requirements. Although I would love to create a personal formula for each of you, I can't do it because I haven't met you and don't know your individual emotional and physical case histories. So, I'm afraid you'll have to do some of the work for yourselves.

Throughout this book I've given 'palettes' of essential oils to choose from. The oils for men and women are often different, and the oils for particular requirements are different. You can create your own masterpiece by choosing oils from one palette or several palettes, depending on the requirements of you or your lover at any particular time. You are aiming to produce a 'portrait in a bottle' that matches the emotional and physical picture of you or your lover.

When making a formula for your lover, try to mix the oils with them, choosing by smell preference and intuition, in addition to the needs and desires identified by the book. If you're planning to create two 'portraits', one for you and one for your lover, compare the oils that you would both like to try, and pick one that appears on both lists. Aim to create harmony between the two of you by including this chosen oil in each formula.

Whether you're using one of my synergistic blends or creating one for yourself, put the various proportions of essential oil all together in a small bottle. You can then take however many drops you need from this bottle for your bath, shower, massage oil or room method as and when required. It's far better to pre-prepare the synergistic blends rather than mix them on the spot, because the molecules of the various components then have a chance to interact with each other and become thoroughly synergized.

The principle of mixing various components together to create a new, harmonious whole is as old as civilization itself. The ancient Egyptians prepared perfumes made from as many as twenty ingredients, and some time around the first century BC a Chinese book was written telling of the exploits of the king, Liu an, who greeted his guests with luxury 'while there was burning the incense of a hundred ingredients, harmoniously compounded'. Beethoven composed musical symphonies by using dozens of instruments, while Leonardo da Vinci created artistic masterpieces by using dozens of colours – all 'harmoniously compounded'.

A synergistic blend, like a Beethoven symphony, is more than the sum of its parts. It is something new, something special. But the gift of creation can be yours, too. You can use the palettes throughout this book, your nose to detect a harmonious aroma, and your intuition. With your love, and with the information in this book, you have everything you need to create your own masterpieces – formulas which are uniquely right for you and your lover!

FUN FORMULAS FOR YOU AND YOUR LOVER

Throughout the text of *Fragrant Sensuality* a choice of essential oils has been given because of several factors. First, smell preference – a valuable indicator in deciding which particular oil or formula to use, because people are actually drawn to the oils with which they are in harmony and which can meet their need. Second, availability – one cannot always find one's first choice of oil; and third, cost. Also, each oil and formula has its own characteristics, and these are very much worth exploring. Lastly, we change, and the choice of essential oils can change with us.

But just suppose that you like the aroma of *all* the oils and they are available and within your price range. Where to start? To answer this question you can turn to the chart on pages 53–55 for clues as to which oils to choose. On the left is the common name of the oil with its Latin name below, from which its number is derived. To the right of that you'll find hair-colour types for the male and female. If you cannot be sure of the colour of your lover's hair, either because it's dyed or because it's gone grey, refer instead to the skin-type chart on page 52. There are four ways to use the chart. First, it can be a simple, extra aid when making a decision about which oil to choose from the main text of the book. Just look up all the oils you're interested in, and compare them to see which most relates to you in terms of number-affinity, and hair and body types.

If you want to examine all the essential oils to find those which most relate to you, cross reference them all. Find your birthdate and name numbers and write down a list of those oils of the same number – this is your number-affinity list. Now go through the whole essential oil chart again, ticking off against your number-affinity list the oils which are also in your hair- and body-type columns. The oil(s) with two or three ticks are most compatible with you, but all the oils on your personal list will be fun choices for you whether used alone or in a personal formula.

You can also make a formula by choosing one oil of number-affinity, and one each from the hair-type and body-type affinity columns. The other deciding factor in this method will be smell preference, which is in itself a good guide to compatibility with yourself.

To make an Aromantic love potion for you and your lover to share, make two lists of number-affinity oils –

one for you and one for your lover. Now go through the chart again, ticking off against the relevant list those oils which are hair- and body-compatible. Start your love potion with an oil that appears on both your lists. Continue to add the oils that seem most compatible – either to you both, or to you individually, and formulate a blend that suits *both* tastes.

Numbers

Numerology is the science of numbers founded by the Greek mathematician and philosopher, Pythagoras. You'll need your lover's exact date of birth, the numbers of which you add together to find a single-digit number. Don't forget the 19 in the year: i.e., don't add 4.7.56, but 4.7.1956. This example would work out as follows:

$$4+7+1+9+5+6=32; \ 3+2=5$$

When finding the number of a name, use the name that the person chooses to call themselves. If your lover was named Archibald Ebenezer Smith by his parents but prefers to be known as 'Ben Smith' (and who can blame him?) then refer to the chart below to arrive at the number 9, as shown underneath the chart.

1	2	3	4	5	6	7	8	9
A	B	C	D	E	F	G	H	I
J	K	L	M	N	O	P	Q	R
S	T	U	V	W	X	Y	Z	

B   E   N   S   M   I   T   H
$2 + 5 + 5 + 1 + 4 + 9 + 2 + 8 = 36; \ 3 + 6 = 9$

If your lover uses an initial for a middle name in correspondence and prefers to see letters addressed to him or her which include the use of this initial, by all means include it in your reckoning. The important thing is to arrive at a number that accurately reflects your lover and that includes how your lover sees themself.

Hair and skin types

It isn't always possible to tell the natural colour of your partner's hair, but you can get some guidance from the complexion of the skin. For example, someone with pale, translucent skin would benefit from oils on the blond hair list. A freckled person would be best suited to the essential oils on the redhead list.

Skin type	Hair list
Fair	Blond
Sensitive	Blond
Translucent	Blond
Freckled	Redhead
Reddish tinge	Redhead
Dehydrated (dry)	Blond
Fragile	Blond
Greasy	Black
Spotty	Black
Normal	Brunette
Oily	Brunette
Oily and normal (combination)	Brunette
Dry and normal	Blond

Body types

The human form grows to all shapes and sizes and it can be useful to take this into consideration when choosing an essential oil. There are basically three types, as classified by anthropologist Dr William H. Sheldon, each having a certain body frame and structure. He devised the terms endomorph, mesomorph and ectomorph.

THE ENDOMORPH. This type of person can be obese or have a tendency to put on weight fast. If a woman, she has rounded hips and thighs and heavy arms and stomach, yet her hands and feet are usually small. Endomorphs diet continuously – but never seem to win the battle! They exercise infrequently and slowly.

THE MESOMORPH. These are the athletic type. They have a muscular frame and usually retain a good figure, but their body can sag if they don't exercise.

THE ECTOMORPH. Ectomorphs are thin and angular. Their body is long and thin and they can usually eat a mountain of food without putting on a gram of weight. If they do gain weight, it's usually on the abdomen.

ESSENTIAL OIL with Latin name	NUMBER	HAIR TYPES (M) MALE/(F) FEMALE				BODY TYPES		
		Blond	Brunette	Redhead	Black	Mesomorph (muscular)	Ectomorph (thin)	Endomorph (rounded)
Ambrette *Hibiscus abelmoschus*	1			M		×		
Angelica *Angelica archangelica*	8			F		×		
Anis vert *Pimpinella anisum*	6	M			×			
Basil *Ocimum basilicum*	1				M			×
Bay *Laurus nobilis*	1				M		×	
Benzoin *Styrax benzoin*	3	M/F					×	
Bergamot *Citrus bergamia*	2		M/F					×
Black pepper *Piper nigrum*	2			M		×		
Bois de rose *Aniba rosaeodora*	3	M				×		
Cardamom *Elettaria cardamomum*	4			M			×	
Cedarwood *Cedrus atlantica*	6				M	×		
Chamomile Roman *Anthemis nobilis*	7	F					×	
Cinnamon *Cinnamomum zeylanicum*	2		M					×
Clary-sage *Salvia sclarea*	7		M/F				×	
Coriander *Coriandrum sativum*	5		F					×

ESSENTIAL OIL with Latin name	NUMBER	HAIR TYPES (M) MALE/(F) FEMALE				BODY TYPES		
		Blond	Brunette	Redhead	Black	Mesomorph (muscular)	Ectomorph (thin)	Endomorph (rounded)
Cumin *Cuminum cyminum*	3		M					×
Cypress *Cupressus sempervirens*	7	F					×	
Fennel *Foeniculum vulgare*	7	F						×
Frankincense *Buswellia thurifera*	3		M				×	
Geranium *Pelargonium graveolens*	4		M/F					×
Ginger *Zingiber officinale*	8			M				×
Grapefruit *Citrus paradisi*	5	F					×	
Hyacinth *Hyacinthus orientalis*	7			F				×
Jasmine *Jasminum officinale*	9	F	F	F	M/F	×		
Lavender *Lavandula officinalis*	7			F				×
Lemon *Citrus limonum*	7				M	×		
Lime *Citrus aurantifolia*	1				F			×
Mace *Myristica fragrans*	3		M				×	
Mandarine *Citrus reticulata*	3			F			×	
Marjoram *Origanum marjorana*	9			F		×		
Melissa *Melissa officinalis*	1			M				×
Mimosa *Acacia decurrens*	8		M			×		
Myrrh *Commiphora myrrha*	5				M		×	
Narcissus *Narcissus poeticus*	6				M		×	

54

ESSENTIAL OIL with Latin name	NUMBER	HAIR TYPES (M) MALE/(F) FEMALE				BODY TYPES		
		Blond	Brunette	Redhead	Black	Mesomorph (muscular)	Ectomorph (thin)	Endomorph (rounded)
Neroli *Citrus aurantium*	1	F					×	
Nutmeg *Myristica fragrans*	4			· F			×	
Orange *Citrus sinensis*	1		M					×
Palma rosa *Cymbopogon martini*	2				M	×		
Patchouli *Pogostemon patchouli*	1			M	F			×
Pettigraine *Citrus aurantium*	1				F	×		
Pimento berry *Pimento officinalis*	3			F		×		
Pine *Pinus sylvestris*	3	M					×	
Rose Bulgar *Rosa Damascena – centofolia*	7	F	F	F	F	×		
Rose Maroc *Rosa Damascena*	6			F	F	×		
Rose Turk *Rosa Damascena – centofolia*	7	F	F				×	
Rosemary *Rosmarinus officinalis*	6				F	×		
Sandalwood *Santalum album*	6	M				×		
Tonka bean *Dipteryx odorata*	6	F						×
Vanilla *Vanilla planifolia*	4				M		×	
Vervaine (verbena) *Lippia citriodora*	4	F				×		
Vetiver *Vetiveria zizanoides*	5		M			×		
Violet leaf *Viola odorata*	5		F				×	
Ylang-ylang *Cananga odorata*	7		F				×	

HOW AND WHERE TO USE NATURE'S ESSENTIAL OILS

The following list is arranged by three methods of use: water, body and room. A full volume-guide for massage oils, giving the minimum and maximum volumes relative to base-oils follows this chart.

The room methods are subtle, so if you remain in the room after preparing it with essential oil, you may find the aroma hardly perceptible, because your olfactory nerves adjust so quickly. (It's just like a smoke-filled room can be very noticeable when you walk into it but you can get used to it quickly.) To judge how powerful the aroma really is, prepare the room with your chosen method, then leave, shutting the door behind you, and return in a few minutes. In this way you'll be able to perceive the aroma clearly and judge the power of the volume you're using. The chapter 'Ambience and the Aromantic Aura' will give you a selection of further methods.

Essential oils are about poetry. Homer recognized this and wrote 'Here first she bathes, and round her body pours; Soft oils of fragrance and ambrosial showers; The winds, perfumed, the balmy gale conveys, Through heaven, through earth, and all the aerial ways.' And Aromantics is about love, so add the thought of it as you prepare your chosen oils and method.

THE METHOD LIST		
WATEMETHODS	DOSAGE	
BATH	As directed in the relevant chapter, or maximum 8 drops	Put the drops on to the surface of the water after the bath has been run. In a few formulas the essential oil is mixed with a little base-oil before it's put on the water. Close the door when you prepare the bath so the vapours don't escape. Soak for at least ten minutes, relax and breathe deeply.
BIDET	As directed or 2–3 drops	Use warm water from the tap. Put the essential oil on to the water after it's been run and swish it around so you don't leave big globules on the surface; they could irritate delicate mucous membranes.

WATER METHODS	DOSAGE	
DOUCHE	Only as directed	Use boiled and cooled water from the tap or bottled spring water which has been warmed. Add the essential oil, filter the mixture through a paper coffee filter, and shake the douche thoroughly.
JACUZZI	3 drops per person	See 'The Other Side', page 219, for the list of essential oils which have antibacterial and antiviral properties and which may offer you protection against bacteria and viruses which may be swimming around with you in communal jacuzzis.
SAUNA	2 drops per pint/560 ml of water	Use eucalyptus, tea tree or pine essential oils. Mix in the water beforehand, and throw water on heat-source as usual. Only use the three suggested essential oils, which are excellent cleansers and detoxifiers. They enter the body with inhalation and expel the toxins by perspiration.
SHOWER	Maximum 4 drops unless otherwise directed	Wash as normal, then add the essential oil to your wash-cloth or sponge, which should be wet, and rub the wash-cloth or sponge all over yourself briskly as you continue to stand under the running water of the shower. Breathe the aromatic steam in deeply through the nose.
SITZ BATH	2–3 drops unless otherwise directed	Run the warm water from the tap into the bath so it's at hip level. Alternatively, lower your derrière into a bowl. Add the essential oil and swish it around with your hand so there are no big globules left on the surface of the water which could irritate the delicate mucous membrane.
BODY METHODS	**DOSAGE**	
INHALED AS A VAPOUR	2–3 drops	Pour hot water into a large bowl, add the essential oil, lean over the bowl with your face about ten inches away, cover your head with a towel and drape it around the sides of the bowl so that no vapour escapes. Close your eyes and breathe deeply through your nose for about one minute.

BODY METHODS	DOSAGE	
MASSAGE OIL	As directed or maximum of 1 drop per 1 ml See chart at end of this section for complete minimum and maximum quantities per different volumes of base-oil	Add the essential oil to a vegetable base-oil – used either singly or mixed: almond, hazelnut, peach kernel, apricot kernel, grapeseed, soya or peanut. To dissolve the oils: add the essential oil to the base-oil in the bottle, turn the bottle upside down a couple of times and then roll the bottle briskly between the palms of your hands. **If you have any allergies** to cosmetics, soaps, perfumes, etc., it is advisable to do an allergy test on a small section of skin twenty-four hours before you plan to massage. The amount needed for a massage can be ascertained by cupping the palm of your hand and putting as much massage oil in as it will hold without spilling over on to the fingers or over the edge of the palm. (The bigger the body to be massaged, the bigger the hand – so that hand is a good gauge of how much is needed.) One teaspoon is quite adequate for most bodies.
TISSUE OR HANDKERCHIEF	1 drop	Just inhale when required.
ROOM METHODS	DOSAGE	
CANDLES	1–2 drops	Light the candle. Wait a while for the wax to start melting, then add the essential oil to the melted wax, being careful not to get the essential oil on to the wick. Essential oils are inflammable, so be careful not to put too much on the candle wax.
DIFFUSERS	1–6 drops	Diffusers are specially made for essential oils. They are made of glass, pottery or metal. Some work by candle and some are plugged into the electricity supply; they gently heat the essential oil, allowing the molecules to rise into the atmosphere of the room.

ROOM METHODS	DOSAGE	
LIGHTBULB	1–2 drops maximum	Put the essential oil on to a lightbulb in a table lamp when the light is off. Be careful that the oil doesn't run down the bulb and into the fitment. It's better to prepare this method with a dropper to make sure you don't use too much. The light can be turned on immediately or up to a week later. Don't put the oil on the bulb when the bulb is already turned on because essential oils are inflammable. There are commercially available products, rings of non-flammable material or metal rings, for using the essential oil with lightbulbs.
RADIATOR OR HUMIDIFIER	1–9 drops	If your radiator has a humidifier attachment, simply add the essential oil to the water. Alternatively, put the essential oil on to a dry cottonwool ball and put it on top of the radiator or lodge it by the pipe. Humidifiers: simply add the essential oil to the water. It takes 5–10 minutes for the aroma to permeate the whole room. Although there is no maximum, remember that high doses can be overpowering.
ROOM SPRAY	4+ drops per half pint/280 ml water	Use a new plant sprayer. Put warm (not boiling) water in, add the essential oil, shake it around a bit. You can spray the room, curtains, cloth-covered furniture, and carpets. Avoid spraying above polished wooden furniture – as you would avoid putting any water on good, wooden furniture.
WATER BOWL	1–9 drops. Replenish as needed	Put boiling water into a small bowl and add essential oil to the strength you desire. Although there is no maximum, remember that high doses can be overpowering. Place anywhere in the room, close windows and doors and allow 5–10 minutes for the aroma to penetrate the whole room.
WOOD FIRE	1 drop on each log	Use cypress, pine, sandalwood or cedar-wood essential oil. Put it on to the wood before placing it in the fire. This can be done immediately before putting the wood into the fire or any time in advance, because essential oil will retain its effectiveness. The essential oil is inflammable so it will help the wood to catch fire.

QUANTITIES FOR BLENDING ESSENTIAL OILS WITH BASE/VEGETABLE OILS					
Number of drops of essential oils Minimum–maximum quantities	Amount of base/vegetable oil				
	Ml	Fl oz	Teaspoons	Dessertspoons	Tablespoons
1	1				
2– 5	5		1		
4–10	10		2	1	
6–15	15	½ (approx.)	3	★	1
8–20	20		4	2	★
10–15	25		5	★	★
12–30	30	1 (approx.)	6	3	2

★ indicates that this becomes a fractional quantity – so use a precise measurement, in teaspoons for example.

The 'Number of drops' indicates the minimum to maximum allowed per measurement, unless otherwise stated in formulas/blends.

Please note: pregnant women should always use the minimum quantities, shown here and in all blends and formulas.

Essential oils will give you approximately twenty drops per ml.

(You can buy oils in quantities right up to one litre.)

3

The Desire For Touch

Just holding hands can be an electrifying experience. Remember young love? Hands held together as if by some magnetic pull, inseparable . . . one unit . . . 'us'. And now, too, I hope, as you and your lover sit holding hands, the flow of energy between you is palpable, not in terms of atoms or words, but clear enough all the same. Touch is a real channel of communication and lovers transmit secret messages and silent poetry through touch.

'To touch' is a verb of possibilities. My thesaurus gives a few, including 'to feel, stroke, squeeze, kiss, caress, fondle, handle, massage, knead, rub, press, pat, tap, lick, brush, flick, tickle, scratch, twiddle' and, would you believe, 'fiddle with'. Need I say more? But touch is also an interface, a link, and the thesaurus again provides the vocabulary: 'To make contact, adjoin and converge.' We're definitely getting there but, as far as sex is concerned, the word 'touch' is, potentially, even more interesting: 'To have an effect upon, influence, inspire, impress, mark, melt, move, soften and stir.' Now we're talking!

Touch is a subject with many aspects. Not all touch is

the same. Even the most common form of social contact – the handshake – is quite different from person to person, and we make quick character judgements based upon it. We note the energy, strength and force of the hand, and feel it to be either cold or warm, damp or dry. This momentary touch can decide whether we want to do business with a person, make love with them, or get as far away from them as possible . . . and it was just one quick touch. They can talk all they want, but we have already made our decision because touch said it all.

Touch is used in many different forms of healing – including acupressure, reflexology, shiatzu, osteopathy or chiropractic, massage in its many forms, and the oldest system of all – 'laying on of hands'. Most therapists can 'read' a body like a book and touch is both a diagnostic and therapeutic form. When in the hands of a qualified remedial therapist, massage has many clinically observed physiological benefits, including the healing of psoriasis and eczema. But the therapeutic benefits of touch could start long before the person becomes a patient, and all studies bear out experience – people deprived of touch suffer in one way or another. On the very simplest physical level, touch stimulates the circulation of blood and this, in turn, stimulates muscle and nerve action. As a vibrant working of nerves and muscles is so important to sexual excitation and response, the importance of touch to Aromantics is obvious. But there is more to touch than this . . .

THE HUNGER FOR TOUCH

The human being thrives on touch. An enormous amount of research has been carried out in recent years, on both human beings and animals, and the results show that its lack ('cutaneous deprivation') can lead not only to emotional disturbances but also to a lessened intellectual ability and physical growth, reduced sexual interest, and even a weakness of the immune system. There are, it seems, distinct biochemical differences between people who experience touch and those who do not.

But, unfortunately, a large number of people go through life with very little tactile stimulation. Over the years in my clinical practice I've met many patients who have little experience of touch. The most worrying aspect relates to self-examination for health reasons – women need to check their breasts for cancer and men need to check for lumps which could indicate testicular cancer. Yet even for such necessary and innocent activities, I've heard patients say, 'Lying there touching myself? I couldn't!'

The connection between sex and touch – any touch – is made early on by many people. The trouble starts when childhood sexuality is controlled by parental admonishments of 'Don't touch yourself!' or 'That's dirty'. 'Good girls don't let boys touch them' is said almost as much as 'Big boys don't cry'. Hugs from strangers, children must be told, are bad.

In one way or another, touch early on can be associated with guilt, and it often becomes acceptable only within the context of secure or 'legitimate' sexual activity. However, this imprisoning of touch within the context of sex means that touch becomes a lead-in to it – 'I know when he wants sex because that's when he puts his arm around me.' Ironically, the end result of this situation is that women often agree to have sex only because they want touch. Sex is the only way they can get the warmth and closeness they need, and many surveys on this subject seem to point to the fact that female promiscuity isn't an insatiable desire for sex, but the hunger for touch.

The hunger for touch is a real human need. It can be difficult for men to admit their need because from the word 'go' they're told to be strong and in control and not to go running to mummy for comfort whenever there's any trouble. The association between weakness and cuddles can easily be transferred into the sexual relationship, so that when the woman attempts to have her hunger for touch satisfied in his arms, he thinks, 'She's being pathetic'. This apparent show of emotional weakness can be especially exasperating for a man who already feels that he is carrying a majority share of the relationship responsibilities. The woman, meanwhile, finds him cold and unresponsive. It is said that women have a better touch than men, if only because it is so much more a part of their daily lives. But because so many people equate touch with sex, these same tactile women may refrain from touching their partners because it will be interpreted as a sexual advance. So for one reason or another, touch isn't always seen as an activity valid in its own right, a legitimate human need, but as a means to an end.

The degree of tactile stimulation in a person's life is very much affected by two things: cultural tradition and family circumstances – the general and the particular. In Japan, until very recently, touching in the street was thought very bad form, while in Italy everyone seems to be touching each other, from children to grannies. In most southern European countries the women walk arm in arm. In Arab and Indian subcontinent countries, men walk holding hands, and mothers massage their babies and children on a regular, almost daily, basis, and are in their turn massaged by them. Only the other day I saw three generations of women from an Indian family stop for a minute at a London shopfront so the granddaughter could massage her grandmother's apparently rheumatic hand. Westerners tend to leave the massaging of grandma's rheumatism to the physiotherapist.

Babies carried in the slings that parents hitch around their chests, so the baby is held close, are far more secure when left with strangers than babies who are transported around in baby buggies. Children are always craving to be touched and hugged, but because mother is so often busy the child often gets rejection instead – 'Don't bother me now'. Yet the need remains, and becomes amplified so that some may be naughty only to get a slap because this touch is better than no touch at all!

Fortunately, a person who has 'lost their touch' is not lost forever. Because I give my patients essential oil treatments to use at home, I often ask the question, 'Have you got someone to massage you – your husband perhaps?' And often the reply is 'Oh no, we never touch', or 'He never has' – and some of these women and men have been married for thirty years or so. (And when was the last time *you* gave or received a massage?) Nevertheless, the patient very often finds the partner willing to take part in the treatment, and I hear enthusiastic reports: 'He's got a lovely touch, you know.' Soon they want to return the compliment and pleasure and start to massage their partner, and a whole new dimension of tactile experience is opened up.

THE AROMANTIC TOUCH

When sexual energy between a couple is high, there's not such a need to 'go all the way' because touch, as an activity in itself, can be a wholly satisfying experience, too. One might not always want to make love, especially after a long and tiring day, but when ten minutes of potentized touch takes place, the same relaxing and satisfying feeling overtakes you and you fall into each other's arms, close and at one instead of grumpy and uptight.

It's crucial to allow yourself to accept that touching doesn't have to lead to sex. Just touch each other in the full knowledge that you're going to fall asleep in ten minutes' time. Caress each other gently, not forgetting the face and head, kiss good night and go to sleep. Sweet dreams.

Three ten-minute, touching-only sessions a week would save thousands of marriages and millions of pounds in psychiatrists' and doctors' fees. First of all, emotional tension is diffused and dispersed so no 'bottling up' occurs. (It's not uncommon for a person to feel close to tears when touched after a long time.) Despite the fact that touch dissolves tension we rarely offer it to people who are 'stressed-out' – cuddles and sympathy are reserved for emotional upsets. If your partner comes home one day in a fury and starts to march around the house sounding off about the day's events, treat them with touch by all means, but make it gradual. Start by taking their hand and simply keep holding it; then stroke their arm. By this time they might have taken a deep sigh and, if you're near a chair, they may be eased into it. Gradually use touch to ease their stress – great demonstrative engulfing embraces at times of high stress can just cause an explosive reaction . . . so gently does it! But we're all subjected to some degree of stress during the day and a ten-minute touching session before sleep can really help to ease the burden.

The human organism is electric and needs earthing. The activity of the brain's 10,000,000,000 nerve cells is mainly electrical, and they interact through the nervous system with the entire body, including the skin. The skin is, in fact, the largest organ of the body. When you gently stroke your lover, you're earthing their electro-magnetic surplus energy, calming the nervous system and helping to balance out the workings of the endocrine system.

With touching, it's as important to have someone who will receive as well as someone who will give – you can't have one without the other. The recipient might look passive, but their energy can be very active! There are two ways to be passive – with a tired listlessness, or with 'purposeless tension', as the ancient Indians would say. It's this second form of passivity that we're trying to aim for here – an alive awareness, relaxed, breathing normally (not held), senses alive, and mentally allowing and encouraging energy flow through the body.

If you have difficulty in accepting passivity you can console yourself with the knowledge that you'll be active when the roles are reversed. But if you find it difficult to accept touch from your lover, you may be in the wrong relationship! All lovers should, at least, be able to happily accept each other and each other's love.

With any form of touch, the most crucial aspect is the thought behind it. Touch is not universally innocent or well meant. Some people touch other people so that they have a surface against which to feel themselves – they aren't concerned about transmitting their love so much as using someone else to create sensation in their own fingertips so that they can love themselves. This is a tricky one, but you'll know it when you feel it. Then there is invasive touch – when someone makes a physical touch to see 'how far they can go'. This is when it's necessary to state an objection to touch with 'How dare you touch me!' so the message gets across that they can't go any further. One doesn't linger over a touch with the boss because it would probably be interpreted as a sexual advance, and for the same reason bosses avoid lingering touches of their female staff. And a punch on the chin is another, more obvious, form of negative touch!

But just as negative thoughts behind a touch can be identified, so too can positive thoughts, which can then be put to good use. One can literally potentize touch with the power of thought. When you touch your lover close your eyes perhaps, but in any event, think of your hands as an extension of your heart – your love – reaching right into their heart through the surface of their skin. Blank out any negativity you may have been feeling through the day towards your lover, just forget about disagreements, put them aside for now and major on the positive – giving love in generosity. If you really concentrate and allow your natural energies and senses to be your guide, your loving touch will become a magnificent and surprising tool which can be incorporated into lovemaking. Touch shouldn't just be a form of foreplay, but an on-going, energy-circulating and stimulating tool, used to fan the fires of passion. Lovemaking is an obvious time to fully utilize the power of touch, if only because this is the only time most of us have our naked skin available, ready and willing. Why waste the chance of taking advantage of it?

Touch can be extremely effective on its own by simply using gentle, stroking movements with the palm and fingers of your hand. Incorporate the well-known erogenous zones of the body – bearing in mind that everyone is unique in this respect – including the neck, ears, shoulders, back, nipples, thighs, buttocks, the curve of the hips, the sides of the body, and not forgetting the feet. There are 72,000 nerve endings in each foot and they're not there for nothing! Try gently stroking, massaging or sucking the feet and toes. No, we're not trying to tickle the partner here; many people experience an exquisite sense of relaxation after a session of foot-attention.

If we accept that touch can be a legitimate activity unrelated to sex, then we can really begin to explore its potential. Our society needs to recognize the beneficial effects touch has on the nervous system with the same readiness as it today pops tranquillizers and sleeping pills. Touch is an important human activity in its own right, crucial to our well-being and an absolute delight. So, let's get in touch!

BIO-MAGNETIC ENERGY

When you touch, the force is with you. You can feel your own forcefield quite easily by forming a closed circuit. Hold your hands at chest level, palms facing each other and about twelve inches apart. The important thing is that your hands are relaxed, so your fingers may be slightly apart and your hands slightly cupped.

When I ask students to do this exercise they invariably tense the fingers, so I repeat: shake your wrists and start again making absolutely sure your hands are completely relaxed – or it simply won't work! Although your whole hands are facing each other, the poles of energy come from the centres of the palms of your

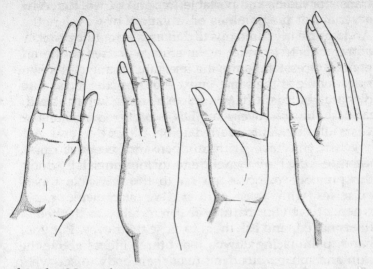

hands. Now, focusing your concentration very slowly bring your hands towards each other until they are about four inches apart and, again very slowly, separate them again to the twelve inches apart position. Move them together and apart like this for about ten minutes and you'll feel the energy build-up between the hands as an elastic, bouncy material, rather like sticky chewing gum. If you do this correctly, you'll also feel a tingling sensation in the backs of your hands which moves to the forearms, the spine, torso, legs and feet, and into the earth.

Although this force is tangible, it remains for a future Nobel Prize-winner to explain what, exactly, it is. Photographs of human energy fields have been taken by researchers at Duke University in America, Dr C. Guja of the Institut V. Babe in Bucharest, Rumania, and students of Dr Kirlian all over the world, amongst others, but there is no certainty that the energy fields they are picking up are one and the same. Indeed, it is more than likely that there are several invisible energy patterns and fields yet to be explained.

Invisibility, as such, should present no barrier to accepting the real – we do, after all, turn on our transistor radios and portable TVs and expect to receive a variety of programmes on a variety of wavelengths. And it is clearly ludicrous to demand 'scientific proof' as a prerequisite to belief when science is itself in the on-going process of disproving itself and changing its own rules, while at the same time extending 'the facts' at its disposal by identifying and explaining what already exists. The 'discovery' of DNA occurred millions of years after DNA first started doing its thing.

When you have, with an open and receptive mind, identified the bio-magnetic energy for yourself by doing the previous exercise, go on to the 'invisible touch' exercises with your partner. We start with 'guess where': have your partner lie comfortably on the bed or floor, naked, and ask them to close their eyes. Put your hand, palm facing down, about three inches above the skin and move your hand over their body to see what energies you can pick up.

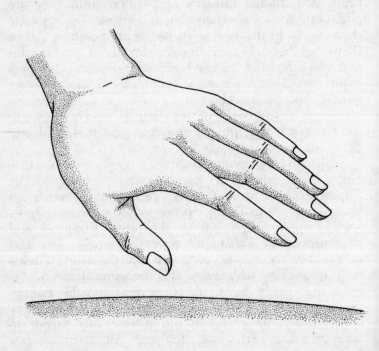

Try to make sure your hand doesn't touch their skin because we want them to say where they feel the hand. When you feel that you've picked up an energy connection stop moving your hand and ask, 'Guess where?'

Closed eyes not only ensure your partner isn't cheating, but make this an act of vulnerability which seems to heighten energy and awareness – perhaps because it necessitates trust! It will be hard for them to resist opening their eyes – but try. You should relax your hand as much as possible without curling the fingers so much that the fingertips touch your partner's skin. Practised couples can achieve obvious and impressive proof of the 'invisible touch' when the partner holds a hand over the man's penis.

For the 'no-touch turn-on', sit or stand opposite each other with your hands outstretched. Each of you turn one hand palm-up and one hand palm-down. You want to match up, palm to palm. Now separate your palms until they're both three inches apart and raise one set of palms about twelve inches above the other.

Right, now you're in position. Relax for a while into the sensation created between the centre of your palms. This is the circuit of feeling created by your two magnetic poles. Build the energy up by slowly moving each pair of hands up and down in opposite directions, as if you were throwing a ball in one hand, and bouncing a ball with the other.

There's no hurry, so just relax into the exercise and enjoy the sensation of the energy flowing between you. Strange as it may seem, this can be a good way to discover new erogenous zones if you let the energy freefall through your body and observe where it goes. Be aware of the areas of energy build-up and make a mental note for future reference. One woman I know discovered an exquisite sensitivity in her buttocks while doing this exercise and now her husband incorporates bottom stroking into their lovemaking – with very sexy results. They'd been married for twelve years and

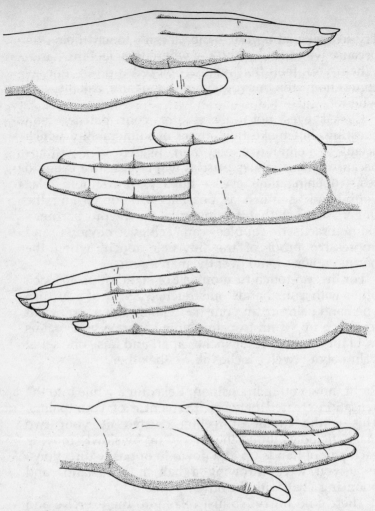

neither of them had realized how important erotic stimulation in this area was to her. Married couples, like scientists, can discover something new every day!

You can, alternatively, mentally direct the energy created by the 'no-touch turn-on' to areas of your body which you already know to be sexually stimulating for you. It may take you both a couple of tries at this exercise for optimum results, but the no-touch turn-on is well worth waiting for!

A bio-magnetic energy build-up can also be easily

incorporated into lovemaking if you sit for five minutes with your backs to each other, naked, about five inches apart, with your eyes closed and your mind concentrating on the space between your backs. You will soon feel the familiar 'bouncy' pull between your two backs. Try consciously to divert this energy to your known erogenous zones. Now, very gently turn towards each other, trying not to break the bio-magnetic connection you have established before boosting the event with sexual intercourse.

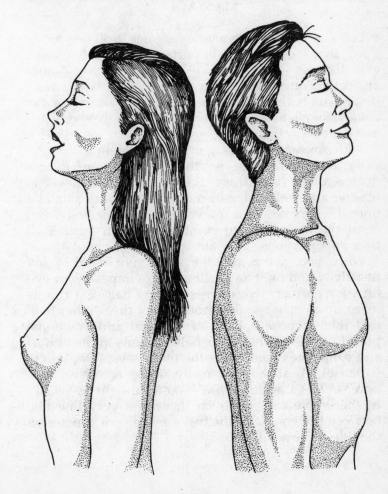

The intimacy of bio-magnetic exchange should be saved for days when your relationship is in harmony. Don't do it if you feel it to be a duty or if either of you is feeling jealous, angry or irritable. Only encourage a profound closeness of this sort when you're in a really positive mood because you're actually sharing and exchanging energy here and neither of you wants to give or receive bad energies.

MASSAGE

When you give an Aromantic massage, you use something that's even more important than your chosen essential oils – your attitude of mind. If you cannot answer the question, 'Do I want this body?' with a yes – don't even bother giving the massage! Wait until a day comes along when you *do* genuinely want that body . . . and then show it.

With Aromantic massage, a sexual feeling, spontaneity and instinct are worth infinitely more than a degree course in massage technique. As you massage, observe and feel the textures of your partner's skin and note the contours and unevenness of their body. But resist the temptation to point out to your partner all their imperfections – they already know all about it!

When you give a massage, clear your mind of any negativity and fight any inclination to impose your ego on your partner. I've often seen one half of a couple jump up to massage the shoulders of their 'other half' and then impose a form of physical and emotional power on them. The 'other half' squirms in discomfort and sometimes pain while the other says, 'Oh, you're so tense'. What they are really saying is, 'Here, look how selfless I am and you, you're uptight as usual'. In the whole area of touch there is a very fine line between the good and the bad – make sure you are on the side of the good!

PREPARING FOR THE AROMANTIC MASSAGE

Choose your massage oil by considering what you're trying to give – relaxation, revitalization or passionate excitation? Look through the chapter that relates to your partner – 'Aromantic man' or 'Aromantic woman'– and discuss between you which formula you want to try.

Now prepare the room. Clear away your lover's business papers or textbooks so they can't catch a glimpse of them out of the corner of their eye and start feeling guilty because they should be working on them. Turn the lights down low or set the scene by lighting a few candles around the room. Use one of the 'room' methods outlined in the Method List to enhance the atmosphere of the room with the particular aura you are trying to create. For this you can use the same essential oil or combination of oils you have chosen for your massage oil, or another, complementary essential oil. Music is a wonderful accompaniment, either gentle and relaxing or heavy rock – you set the scene, so you choose the score.

If you intend to give the massage on the bed, a large towel will protect your sheets from the massage oil. If you're giving the massage on the floor, make sure it will be comfortable – with a big towel on top of a blanket, or whatever. Have ready a couple of small handtowels to lay on your partner as you massage. When you put oil on to one area of their body, you'll need to cover it with a towel to stop the essential oil evaporating, allowing it to sink into the dermis and do its wonderful work. Having these small towels laid on the body also serves to keep your partner warm and alleviates any feeling of vulnerability.

By now the cat will be wandering around, trying to figure out what's going on. It's up to you, of course, but it may be better to put the cat outside – we don't want any distractions. As your last move, take the phone off the hook. The very act of preparation helps to bring your mind into a concentrated, calm frame, simply because you're focusing your energies to one, single aim – providing your lover with an Aromantic touch of love.

When you're giving the massage, make sure you're wearing clothing which is loose around the arms (if, indeed, you're wearing any clothing) because your arms can easily get tired if they're fighting against constricting materials, taking the pleasure of giving the massage away from you, when, and never more so than now, it should be 'as good to give as to receive'!

THE GESTURE OF MASSAGE

When you give the massage, put your body weight behind the movements, flowing with your body. Unless otherwise directed, always move in the direction of the heart: hand to shoulder when massaging the arms; ankle to thigh when massaging the legs; buttocks to shoulder when massaging the back; and when doing the breast or chest area, upwards towards the neck or outwards towards the shoulders. When massaging the stomach, go in a clockwise, circular movement.

This isn't a therapeutic massage, so ignore the images you might have seen in the movies of tough, Scandinavian–style 'chopping' and instead use the more gentle movements outlined below. Creating a balance is important in any massage, so if you massage one arm or leg, make sure you do the other. As you move around the body you can spend a few moments paying special attention to the sexy stimulation points described in the next section, all the while flowing with your intuition, in touch with your partner.

EFFLEURAGE is stroking. These can be long or short strokes, firm or gentle, and these movements are more or less the basic components of sensual massage. Use the whole hand, firmly but relaxed.

Effleurage relaxes muscles which are contracted, strained or tense. Depending on the force behind the movement, the effect on the nerve endings on the surface of the skin can be soothing or stimulating. It can have a deep relaxation effect.

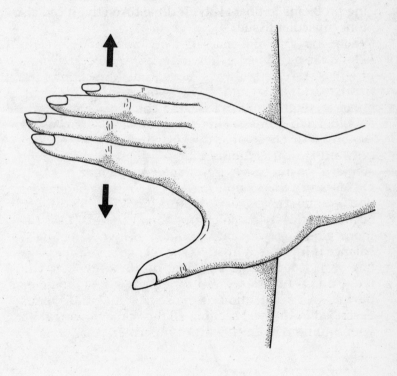

PETRISSAGE also uses the whole hand, although it's more like the action of kneading dough. The movements are firm but never painful – slowly and carefully is the order of the day (or night!). Buttocks respond well to this type of massage.

Petrissage relaxes the muscular tissue leading to an increase in blood circulation and lymphatic flow. As a strong erection depends upon blood flow, the benefits of this type of massage are obvious! Petrissage reduces fatigue by helping to remove lactic acid from the muscles while relaxing hard, contracted muscles, allowing problems to float away. If done correctly, it can also tone muscular tissue.

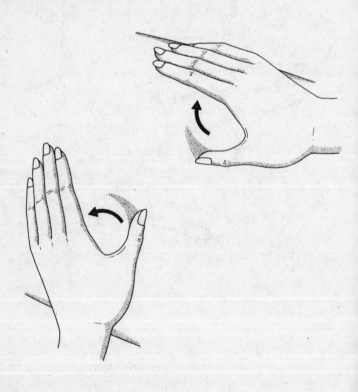

VIBRATIONS are trembling movements. They can be done by either using the middle finger, the forefinger or thumb. The movement is a very light, fast tremble, and you'll find it easier to achieve this if you locate the source of the tremble in your wrist or elbow, rather than in the finger or thumb itself. Vibrations can be done on one spot or along a line on the body. These are particularly good movements to use on the sexy stimulation points which follow.

Traditionally, vibration movements are used to stimulate and alleviate congestion in nerve pathways. Again, this relieves tension and relaxes the person being massaged.

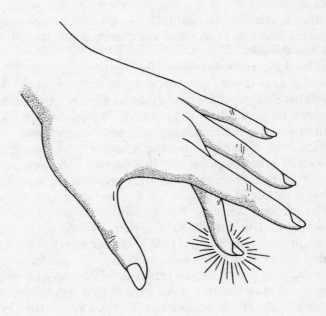

There are many specialized hand movements in massage, like 'frictions', 'clapping', 'hacking' and 'pounding', but they are somewhat vigorous and most people find them inappropriate preludes to making love.

THE SEXY STIMULATION POINTS

If this section were to rely on Western knowledge for its information, the sexy stimulation points would consist of the clitoris and nipples for women, and the penis for men. And what a short section it would be!

But there is also the East. You've probably seen one of the type of kung-fu movies where knowledgeable, oriental people disarm or incapacitate their opponents by the deft application of pressure on one of the body's hidden pressure points. The secret of success is knowing where to press. This is also true for sex, but we are less aware of this aspect of Eastern knowledge simply because while violence is a very public affair, sex is a very private one. But what our kung-fu heroes do behind closed doors (or paper shutters) can be even more impressive than their antics on the street!

The East operates in a different dimension to the West – and it isn't just geographical. Eastern medical systems recognize a whole system of energy lines which cannot be identified as known, physical matter. Acupuncture calls these energy lines 'meridians'. The efficacy of acupuncture simply cannot be denied, so Western sceptics point out that some (and only some) pressure points correspond with physical nerve routes. This is rather like insisting on the existence of a railway network but denying the existence of air lanes and holding up the 'proof' that the two systems are one and the same by pointing out that some airports occur at the same location as some railway stations – *ipso facto*, they are one and the same. To this, the Eastern doctor might reply, 'But wouldn't you *expect* two transportation systems to cross somewhere?' However, the exact reasons for the undisputed effects produced by stimulation of the body's 'invisible wiring system' isn't really our concern here. What matters is that it works. But the air transport analogy is useful because we'll be stimulating areas of the body that are a very long way away from the final destination we want to reach, just as we get on a plane on one side of the globe and get off at the other side!

The following sexy stimulation points include those at the top of the head and the soles of the feet – and all points between. This is *your* journey, however, so make as many stops as you like, or as few. Think of them as pleasant stopping-off points as you journey across your partner's body . . . revitalizing interludes!

The Aromantic massage is an erogenous act and the points shouldn't be pressed in a clinical, curative way, nor, indeed, should you force your ego on your partner by pressing hard. The word to keep in mind is 'gentle'. Incorporate stimulation of the sexy points into your massage by simply paying these areas a little special attention as you come to them, pressing the points gently for a few seconds and then sensitively rubbing the whole area. In some instances I've given instructions for a particular massage technique to be used on the area instead. Try to keep your hand–body contact maintained throughout the massage.

Between them, these sexy points stimulate the sexual organs, blood circulation, and hormone-producing glands. Incorporated into an Aromantic massage, you'll be heightening sexual vibrancy, sensitivity and response.

We start with some points for men, then women, followed by some sexy stimulation points we share. Bon voyage!

For Aromantic Man . . .

Because the area between the navel and pelvic bone is so 'action packed' perhaps the best approach is to treat points **1–3** as a single unit. (Unless you are a skilled therapist!) using the movement to the right, move your thumb upwards in small, round movements, over and over again for a minute or two – with a sexual energy behind the movement!

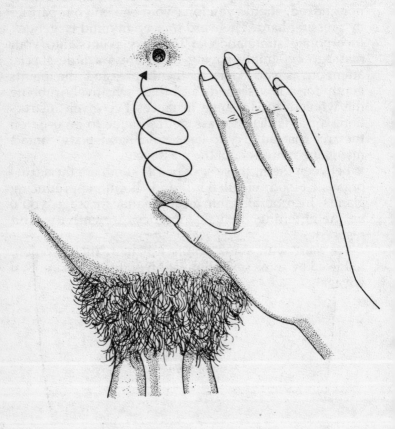

1   *For impotence: halfway between the pubic bone and navel.*
2   *For impotence and premature ejaculation: the point 'Kuan-yuan' – three inches below the navel.*
3   *For premature ejaculation: the point 'Chung-chi' – four inches below the navel, on the upper part of the pubic bone.*
4   *Prostate and testosterone stimulator: on the front – on the lower part of the pubic bone, both sides of the top of the penis. On the back – two inches above the coccyx, on both sides of the crease of the buttocks.*

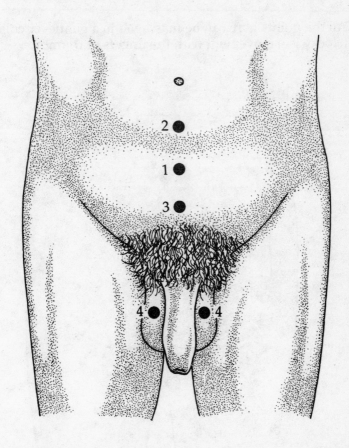

5 *Testosterone stimulator: at the top of the sacrum bone on either side.*

6 *The magic button! Level with the navel, but in the middle of the back.*

7 *(Not illustrated): the point midway between the scrotal sack and the anus. As this is sensitive mucous membrane, you should be very careful to ensure that any massage oil used here is made up according to the instructions in 'The masterly stroke' section (page 203), or that it's stimulated when no massage oil is on your hand.*

All the points here can be massaged in a gentle, circular (clockwise) movement with the fingers or thumbs.

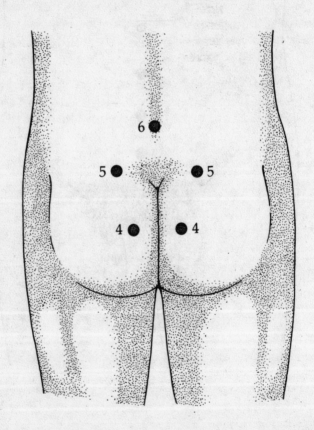

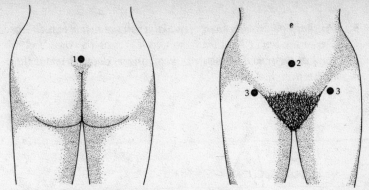

For Aromantic woman . . .

1 *Heightens sexual response: about two inches above the crease of the buttocks.*

2 *Boosts sexual energy and stimulates the vagina: about two inches above the pubic bone.*

3 *Ovaries and uterus stimulator: on both sides where the leg creases, shown here at the upper end of the hairline. But as all women are different, the points may be below the hairline.*

4 *Sexual response and stimulation: on the 'head line' of both hands, where the third finger bends to touch the palm (this can give a whole new dimension to holding hands).*

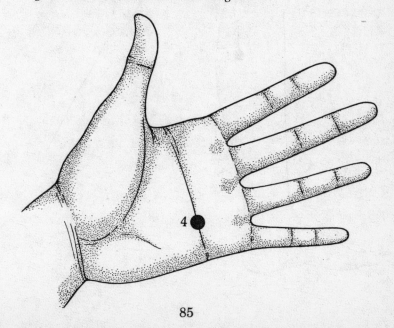

5 *Pituitary point – hormone stimulator: on the inside of both legs. Locate the top of the tibia bone which is near the knee, feel the bend in the tibia and then run your fingers down to about three inches from this point.*

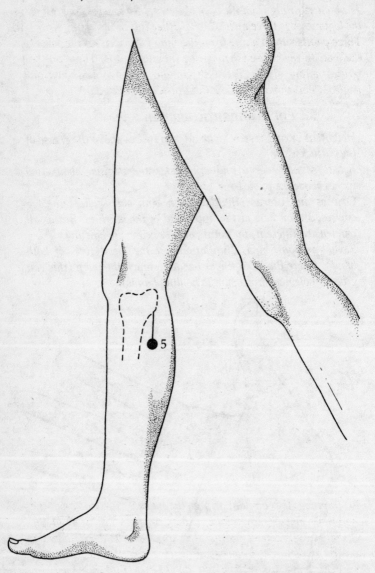

For Aromantic men and women . . . erotic trigger points

1 *The big toes: massage with thumb and fingers.*

2 *The bone running from the back of the heel up towards the calf of the leg: massage three inches along either side of the bone.*

3 *Three points run in a line from the end of the heel, on the sole of the foot, to the crease (shown), by the middle toe. These can be treated as one single line with circular massage as shown on page 82. Fourth point on sole, just inside the bridge.*

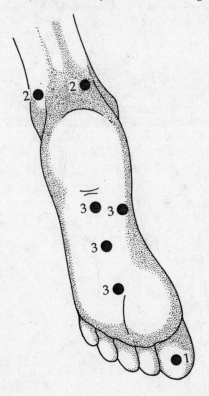

4 *To improve the circulation of the sexual system: use the vibrations massage technique, shown on page 79. Start at the nipple, gently, exerting greater pressure on the shoulder, down the forearm, finishing the movement at the end of the middle finger. See over. If massaging a woman, do not press into the breast.*

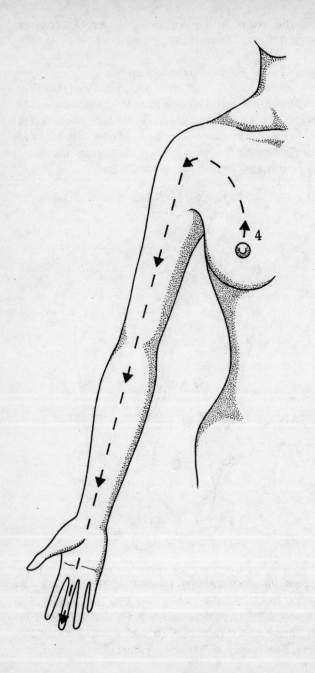

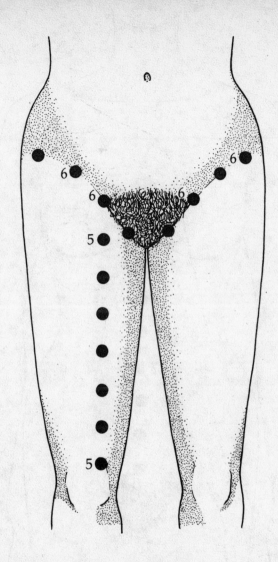

5 *From the top of the leg to the top of the kneecap, on the inner side. Use effleurage or small, circular movements.*

6 *Working on both sides at the same time, use the thumbs in a circular movement, moving outwards along this line and over the hips. Bring your hands over the buttocks and repeat the movement. Don't press into the skin too hard.*

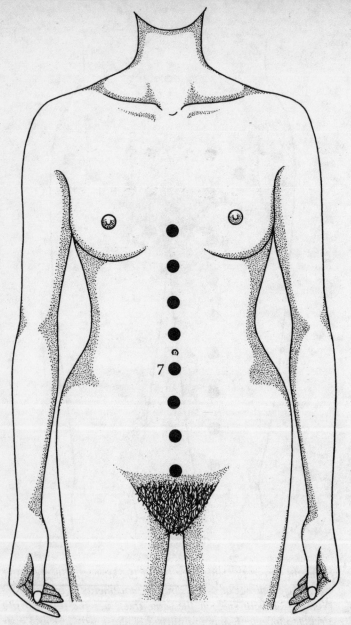

7 In a line moving upwards from the pubic bone to the ribcage, use small, circular movements with the thumb.

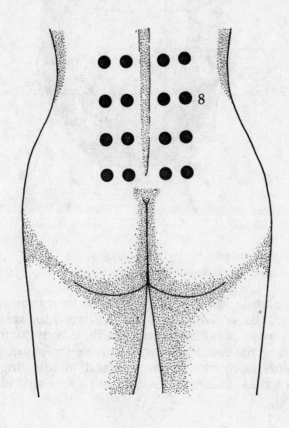

8 *Start either side of the spine, by the crease of the buttocks, moving upwards to above waist-level. Then move your fingers or thumbs out an inch on either side and work up again. Do this complete movement a few times as this is an action-packed area! Use gentle presses, vibrations or circular movements with your thumb or finger.*

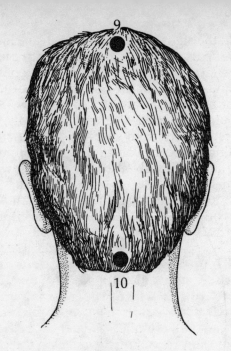

9 *Right at the centre of the top of the head.*
10 *At the centre of the base of the skull.*

Your partner will have to be lying on their front for you to reach these two points. You will need to exert equal pressure so it is best to straddle their body, with your knees on the bed. Press each point gently for a couple of seconds using the forefingers and middle fingers of both hands. Release pressure, wait a few seconds, and repeat.

AROMANTIC MASSAGE

We've already run through most of the points to remember when preparing for a massage – like taking the phone off the hook – but what about romance? The *Kama Sutra* knew what that was: 'The main room should be balmy with rich perfumes and contain a bed, soft, agreeable to the sight, covered with a clean cloth, low in the middle part, having garlands and bunches of flowers upon it, a canopy above it, and two pillows, one at the top and another at the bottom. There should also be a sort of couch, and at the head of this, a stool on which should be placed fragrant ointments, perfume and flowers.' Apart from creating a pleasant atmosphere, setting the scene concentrates the mind, focuses the energy and establishes the mood. It is well worth taking a little time.

You need no specialist techniques to do an Aromantic massage – your greatest asset now is your intuition. You probably already know certain places your lover likes to be touched so spend time incorporating that into your massage. It's up to you whether you want to incorporate 'The sexy stimulation points' or the bio-energy exercises into your massage. The most important thing is to do what your partner likes and wants and, also, what you want. All too often the person being massaged will take the proceedings over. Don't allow this to happen. You are not a slave, but an equal. If your partner wants you to massage a particular place, perhaps in a particular way, and you feel like doing it, fine. If you don't – don't. You have the final say.

Having already decided which oil you are going to use and made it up, ask your partner to lie on their stomach, with the head turned to the side. Their arms can be in any position that feels comfortable so long as they're relaxed. As far as you possibly can, try to maintain some skin contact at all times and keep the movements flowing.

Applying your Aromantic massage oil couldn't be simpler. First pour it on to your own hands; your hands are the method used to apply the massage oil all over your partner's body. Use gentle sweeping movements and make sure the body has a fine sheen to it before you start. If you need to add a little more oil on the body, do so, but remember never to pour the oil directly on to the body. Always pour a little on to your hands and smooth over the areas that feel dry.

Head

1 Using your fingertips massage the head in small circles. Make sure you only use the tips of your fingers and not your nails. The movements should be small, firm and slow. Take your time.

Neck

2 Slide both hands down either side of the neck until the hands are resting on your partner's shoulders. Now turn your attention to the uppermost side of the neck. With both hands, one hand following the other, stroke downwards with slow, loving strokes, reaching to the shoulder. Then gently move the head to the other side and repeat the movement.

Shoulders and Arms

3 Using both hands, slide the hands out towards both shoulders, then down both arms, to the elbow. Use a smooth, firm, slow movement. Now, barely touching, come back up the arm – to the shoulder. Repeat to the elbow two or three times, and then take the movement right down to the hands, returning to the shoulders with the barely touching stroke. Do this whole cycle as many times as you wish.

Back

4 Move your hands to the large (trapezium) muscle which is either side of the vertebrae at the top of the shoulder. With a hand on each shoulder slowly circle the muscles – using gentle but firm movements, utilizing the whole of the hand, in outward, round movements. See page 95. Gradually work your way down to the waist.

5 Return to the shoulders. Using one hand after another, working downwards, your hands vertical with the spine, firmly smooth (on one side) the space between the spine and the shoulder-blade, as if smoothing out the flesh. Now do the other side. Do this movement several times on both sides.

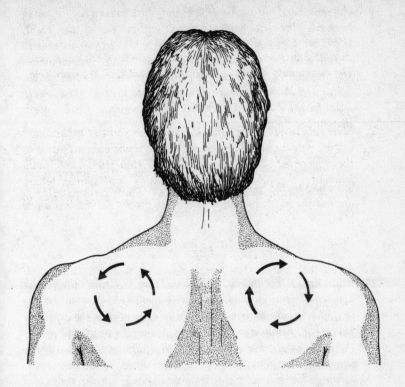

6 *We are now going to massage the waist and lower area but before doing so I just want to say that, as far as Aromantic massage is concerned, the body should be seen as a whole and not as individual portions. Therefore, occasionally return to the upper portion of the body, stroking the back, shoulders and sides when you are predominantly working on the lower part – the object being to draw the whole body energy together.*

7 *Keeping one hand always on the body, alternately stroke from the spine, over the hip, cupping around the side of the body, feeling the pelvic bone. This area is colloquially known as 'the love handles'. Do one side and then the other.*

8 *Using the same movement – both hands alternately stroking – massage the buttocks, wrapping your hands over the hip bone. Do one buttock/hip at a time.*

9   Put one hand on each buttock and start massaging in small circles – the left hand working anti-clockwise; the right, clockwise. Gradually increase the size of the circular movement – and also the movements can become more pronounced – starting gently and becoming firmer. Remember to include the fleshy part in the movement, in other words lifting the buttocks away from the thigh. Eventually the movements should appear like one big circular movement.

10   Now is a good time to bring the upper part of the body back into the massage, as per the point I made in number 6, by sweeping up the back with flat hands, down the side of the body, around the buttocks again, and up the back. Repeat this a few times.

Legs

11   Move now to the thighs, massage one leg at a time. Place your hands on either side of the top of the thigh, just under the buttocks. Avoid touching the genitals, especially the scrotum. Using both hands at the same time, one on the inner and one on the outer thigh, use a movement that lifts and presses at the same time. Very gradually move down the leg to the knee; then, keeping skin contact only, slide your hands up the thigh and repeat twice.

12   Still working on the same leg, repeat the above movement on the calf muscle, working downwards to the ankle. Repeat twice again.

13   Carry out numbers 11 and 12 on the other leg.

Whole Body Sweep

14   Now we have a large sweeping movement which some people find very erotic. Start with your hands on both ankles. Sweep up the inner legs, avoid the genitals and go over the buttocks; sweep up the whole back, to the very top of the neck, over the head, down the side of the head, over the shoulders, down the arms, hands and fingers, back up the inner arms to the armpits, down

*the sides of the body to the feet. Repeat twice, finishing the last
sweep at the shoulders.*

15 *Keeping body contact, move yourself around so that you are at
the top of your partner's head. Now, using the whole hand but
predominantly the fingertips, sweep down the back, either side
of the vertebrae, over the buttocks and up the sides of the body,
pulling slightly as you go. Repeat twice. End this movement at
the head.*

16 *Using both hands, in firm strokes, move over the head, down the
spine – either side of the vertebrae – over the buttocks and into
the inner thighs, down the inner legs, up the outer legs, up the
side of the body, into the underarms, down the inner arm, up the
outer arm, over the shoulders and up to the head again. Repeat
twice.*

Ask your partner to turn over so they're lying on their back.

Head

17 *Massage the head in small circles using the tips of your fingers.
The movements should be small, firm and slow. Take your time.
Be careful not to pull the hair.*

Face and Neck

18 *With one firm, sweeping movement, with your hands on either
side of the face, slowly come down each side of the face, down the
neck, across the collarbone area, over the shoulders and back up
the sides of the neck. Repeat twice. End with your hands on the
temples.*

19 *Turn the hands so they are horizontally across the forehead, one
in front of the other. Using them alternately, stroke upwards
towards the hairline. Continue this movement in smaller
strokes, around the side of the forehead including the temples.*

20 *Now start to think gentle! Move down to the eyes and circle
them with the middle finger of both hands. Be careful not to drag*

the skin under the eye as this is very delicate. Also incorporate the bridge of the nose and the eyebrows, working outwards towards the temples. Repeat several times.

21 Using three fingers on either hand, smooth and lift the cheek muscles gently moving outwards. This movement will end at the temples. For the next part position your fingers under the cheekbones, finishing the movement at the ears. Next, position the fingers slightly below, again moving outwards, this time finishing at the earlobes. The last segment of this movement starts with the fingers in the middle of the chin, along the jaw bone and up to the earlobe. Repeat several times.

Ears

22 Standing at the top of the head, now massage the earlobes, between the thumb and index finger as if you are rolling around small balls. Then massage the whole outer rim of the ear. Do this very gently. Again, repeat several times.

23 Repeat number 18.

Body Sweep

24 Using firm stroking movements, slide the hands down the centre of the body to just above the pubic hairline. Then move the hands out to the hips and sweep back up the sides of the body (on both sides). Repeat twice.

Abdomen

25 Move yourself to the side of your partner's body. Using the whole of your hand massage over the stomach in a clockwise direction. Cover the area from the hairline to the chest, i.e., over the ribcage – the upper and lower abdomen.

Legs

26 Now we are going to massage the legs. Do one complete leg before doing the other. Using two hands at a time, alternately use firm, stroking, upward movements on the outer and inner thigh, working from the knee upwards. Then move to the ankle, and again using the same movements, work upwards to the knee. Do this several times. Then massage the other leg.

27 Holding both legs at the same time, sweep down the entire length of the leg – going down on the outside and up on the inside leg. Repeat several times. Avoid the genitals. End at the waist, by stroking the outer thigh and hips, with an inward movement.

Feet

28 Keeping body contact, move to the feet. Massage one foot at a time. You can hold the foot steady with the other hand, if you wish. Start by massaging the whole of the sole of the foot using the thumb. Then massage each toe with the thumb and the index finger. Lastly, sweep down the feet to the toes, and massage both the top and the sole of the foot. Now do the other foot.

29 For the last movement, use your intuition, stroking or touching your partner in whichever way you and they please.

Seven Important Points To Know Before Starting The Aromantic Massage

1 Unless otherwise stated, the exercise should be repeated twice – i.e., each movement should be done three times in total.

2 Unlike most other massages, the Aromantic massage is solely designed to release sexual vibration and bring electromagnetic harmony between you both. It does this partly by lowering blood pressure and pulse rate. Because the purpose of this massage is so unique, we break away from the usual rule of massage – always going in the direction of the heart. According to the Eastern schools of massage, it increases sensitivity and sensuality in the giver, as well as the receiver. The unique nature of this massage will often bring your breathing into synchronization – that is to say, you will find that you and your partner inhale and exhale at the same time, at the same pace.

3   Throughout this massage your fingers, hands and arms should always be relaxed. They should never be stiff and unyielding; instead you should be following the contours of the body. The simple rule is: the hand yields to the body, not the body yielding to the hand.

4   Whichever Aromantic massage blend of oils you decide to use, it should never be applied directly on to the skin. Pour it into your hands first, then apply. The usual rule is to use an amount between a teaspoon and dessertspoon depending on the size of the body. The amount per person is easily arrived at when we pour our own oil as we cup our hand and use as much oil as the palm of our hand – which is relative to our body size – can hold. But when we massage another person, we don't have this built-in measurement system. As a guide, a woman of average frame will need one teaspoon for each half – front and back – while the average man requires one dessertspoon. Apply the oil before starting the massage and give it a little time to absorb into the body. Apply your teaspoon or dessertspoon or whatever, to your partner's back before starting the back massage; and the same amount to the front of the body before massaging there. The oil should make the body silky and smooth, not oily and slippery.

5   Because this massage is designed to harmonize energies and release sexual vibration, to interrupt it by touching the genitals will somewhat defeat the purpose of the exercise. What genital touching tends to do is dissipate the energy at this stage; it also leaves the partner in a state of suspended tension. Try to get to the end if you can!

6   If your partner is a woman, don't massage her breasts. Obviously your hands will be passing over her breasts and you will be touching them, but breasts are delicate and really don't need massaging as such.

7   This massage is not intended as a prelude to lovemaking, it can be seen as an activity complete within itself. It will certainly bring you into bio-magnetic harmony which is, itself, a wonderful buzz.

THE TEN-MINUTE SELF-MASSAGE

You do not have to carry out this complete massage. Do as little or as much as you like, and take as little or as long as you like to do it – that might be less or more than ten minutes. The title 'Ten Minutes' just gives you a guide as to how long it will take once you have the movements memorized. By all means extract from the total massage those particular sections you're interested in at any particular time – you might want to massage your head after a long tiring day at the office, for example, or massage your tummy and hips with the PMS oil before your period. This massage is suitable for either men or women.

When preparing your massage oils you can also prepare a face massage oil for your facial skin type. You can use the facial massage section separately and benefit each day from the rejuvenating qualities the essential oils have.

Skin Types

Dry .... Sandalwood, Rose
Sensitive .... Chamomile, Lavender
Oily .... Lavender, Ylang-ylang
Normal .... Geranium, Neroli

Dilute 15 drops of your chosen essential oil in 30 ml
of almond oil

1   *Prepare your massage oils.*

Head and Face

2   *Using your fingertips, massage all over your scalp in small circles, firmly but gently.*

3   *Pour a little face oil on to your hand – don't use too much or it won't soak into your skin. Cover your face and neck with the oil.*

4   Alternately, using the heels of your hands, smooth upwards from the centre of your forehead, towards the hairline.

5   Using the fingertips of both hands at the same time, starting just above the eyebrows and moving outwards towards the hair, press and release. Now do this same movement, slightly above, moving upwards in this fashion, covering the whole forehead.

6   Using both hands, take the eyebrow between your index finger and thumb, and press. Start at the bridge of the nose, moving outwards in small segments – about 6–8 in all.

7   Using both hands, squeeze the cheek muscle between the thumb and forefinger. The thumb should be below the muscle, and the forefinger above. They should both be horizontal to the face. Start either side of the nose and work outwards towards the ears. (All face massage should move in this outwards direction, which helps to 'lift' the face.)

8   Using the same pinching movement, go around the chin, starting in the centre and working outwards towards the ears.

9   With your two forefingers, press above the upper lip. Start in the middle and work in an outwards direction. Then repeat the movement under the lower lip.

Neck

1   Clasp both hands over the back of your head and with your thumbs firmly massage the base of your skull, pressing each segment in turn. Start in the middle and work outwards.

2   If lack of mobility prevents you using movement number 1, substitute movement number 2. If you can manage number 1, also do number 2. Place both hands behind your head, approaching under the ears. Massage along the hairline, using the fingers of both hands in small circular movements, quite firmly. Work from the middle outwards.

3   Place your fingers under the skull at the back and, using the fingers of both hands massage in small circular movements. Start this movement on either side of the bone, moving downwards. Now move your fingers slightly further away from the bone, and again repeat the movements, massaging downwards. Continue massaging outwards until the whole neck has been covered.

4   Using one hand at a time, clasp the back of your neck firmly and squeeze. Work from top to bottom. Repeat with the other hand.

Ears

1   Massage both earlobes between your thumbs and index fingers, in circular movements, as if you were rolling small balls between your fingers.

2   Massage the outer rims of the ears in the same manner.

Shoulders

Now change to your body oil, pour a small amount into your hand and apply all over your shoulders, chest and arms. It is easier when massaging yourself to apply the oil at each section of the massage.

1   Reach one arm across the front of your body until you can grip the opposite shoulder muscles. Lift and squeeze the flesh and muscles – as much as you can even if they feel tight. Start by the neck and work outwards. Repeat on the other side.

2   From the above position, massage in this same manner – the whole shoulder, extending downwards to the T-shirt sleeve line. Repeat on the other side.

Hands and Arms

1   Resting the back of your hand on your knee, massage the fingers by gently pressing and stretching them in turn.

2   *Now rest the hand on the palm of your other hand and massage the palm with your other thumb; use small circular movements over your whole palm.*

3   *Stroke up the inside of the arm to the armpit.*

4   *Stroke up the outside of the arm to the elbow. Then squeeze the muscles in the top of the arm, using the whole hand. Try to cover the whole of the top of the arm.*

5   *Repeat all the above on the other side.*

Chest

1   *With two or three fingers of your left hand, press and release slowly and in small portions, nudging along the top of the collarbone, to the right shoulder. Repeat this movement under the collarbone, this time ending close to the armpit.*

2   *Again starting in the centre of your body, do the same movement across the chest to the armpit. Repeat once again, moving downwards each time. When you reach the breast, stop.*

3   *Repeat numbers 1 and 2 on the other side.*

4   *Starting in the centre of the breastbone, just under the level of the collarbones, press into the skin and release using all the fingers of both hands. Massage down to where the ribcage separates. Now continue this press-and-release movement under the ribcage, on either side, until you reach the sides of your body. Carry out this movement slowly.*

Abdomen

Apply the body oil to your abdomen in a clockwise direction and smooth the oil over the hips and buttocks.

1   *Lock the fingers of both hands together and press your hands against your body, just under the breast. Now, with a firm*

104

movement, sweep across your body, left to right and back again. Slowly work downwards until you reach the pelvic bone.

2   *With the same clasping/locked finger position, massage over the whole of the abdomen in a clockwise circular movement.*

3   *Use the same movement as above, this time in the area between the navel and the pubic bone, extending as far as you can over the hips.*

Hips and Buttocks

1   *Using both hands at the same time, place each hand on a buttock and sweep them up the cleavage, over the hips, down the front of the body (no further to the centre than your hands would ordinarily hang if relaxed), around the hips again to the buttocks and over the hips again to the front.*

2   *Form your hands into fists and reach behind your back. Use the knuckles to massage in small circular movements that area known as the sacrum. This is the hard, bony part at the bottom of your spine.*

3   *Using one hand now, still in a fist, massage with your knuckles – starting at the sacrum, moving over the hip, following the pelvic bone until it disappears in the front. Repeat on the other side.*

Back

Apply the oil to as much of your back as you can reach, also your hands. As you are carrying out the movement the oil will spread itself over your back.

1   *Using both hands, again in the fist position, massage with your knuckles up the spine from the sacrum, as far as you can reach. You can use one hand at a time, but it's easier with two. You may find that you are more agile on one side than the other but don't worry, this often improves with the massage.*

Cool Out

1   With your right hand reach across to your left shoulder and
    squeeze the large muscle that lies on the shoulder, close to the
    neck, slightly to the back. Squeeze between the whole hand for a
    count of five; release for a count of three; squeeze again – three
    times in total. Repeat on the other side.

2   Tip your head to the left, to the right, to front, and back. Each time
    leave the head until it has relaxed and fallen as far as it will go.

3   Stretch your right arm high into the air as far as you can, then
    stretch your left arm.

Legs

Apply the body oil to your legs and feet smoothing
upwards.

1   Using both hands on one leg, sweep firmly up the leg from ankle
    to knee. For this movement your thumbs should be at the front
    and your fingers to the back. With the sweep, press your
    fingertips into the calf muscle.

2   Carry out this same movement on the thigh, knee to hip.

3   Using both hands alternately, starting at the knee, take as much
    outer thigh flesh as you can grasp in your hands and squeeze.
    Move slowly upwards towards the hip, squeezing and letting
    go, one hand following the other.

4   Use the same movement but on the front of your thigh; then the
    inner thigh and lastly the back of the thigh.

5   Place one hand between the legs and under the knee and the
    other under the knee but approaching from the outer side.
    Smooth upwards and across the top of the leg in a diagonal
    movement. Now use both hands to sweep the inner thigh, again
    in this diagonal, alternate movement, working from knee to hip.
    Repeat this movement on the outer part of the leg.

6 *Repeat numbers 1–5 on the other leg.*

Feet

1 *Put your left foot on your right knee. With the fingers of your left hand clasped over the top of your left foot, and your left thumb resting on the middle sole of your left foot, your right hand holding your toes, gently massage with your left thumb all over the sole of the foot. Don't forget the area where the toes meet the foot, and the instep, and the heel.*

2 *Still in the same position, using the thumb and forefinger of your right hand, massage each toe in turn. It's as if you're rolling the toes between thumb and forefinger. Do this quite firmly.*

3 *Repeat on the other foot.*

Cool Out

Stretch your legs, pointing your toes like a dancer, stretching one leg at a time. Next, stretch your left arm high into the air, as far as you can. Then stretch your right arm, and relax completely, breathe deeply several times.

4

Aromantic Woman

HOW TO BECOME THE AROMANTIC WOMAN

A woman these days is expected not only to look great and keep the house looking like a colour spread in *Interiors* magazine, but to follow a career, be financially independent *and* bring up the children to be all-round Fabulous Human Beings. We might have won the right to freedom and choice, but our prize was extra work!

As modern women have so many demands upon their time, energy and personal resources, is it any wonder that so many are sitting at the doctor's, waiting for the next prescription of tranquillizers? That is, of course, if they aren't sitting there waiting for the latest prescription to solve one of the innumerable gynaecological problems. 'I just wish my boyfriend could go through one day of a really heavy, painful period,' a young woman I know hissed through her teeth, '. . . just one day.' Well, it isn't just one day for us but about two and a half thousand days over forty years, plus the days of premenstrual tension, menopause flushes, pelvic imflammatory pain . . . and all the rest.

The formulas in this chapter will not only help with a few female reproductive problems, but will also make you into an Aromantic woman.

The Aromantic woman radiates well-being and self-confidence. She has about her the air of a woman loved and in love: she looks fabulous and feels as if she could do anything – singing and whistling as she goes. Nothing negative seems to touch her; everything in the world is wonderful. Men suddenly seem to notice her; she exudes a vibrancy that is unmistakable and irresistible.

You can be the Aromantic woman wherever you are. A body oil applied in the morning will be working all day. At the office, use the water-spray or water-bowl method. On the bus, pull out your Aromantic tissue when the hurly-burly threatens to overwhelm you, and when you get home put a couple of drops of your favourite oil – or synergistic blend of oils – on to a light-bulb or other heat source, and let the molecules gently drift around your home as you unwind and rediscover your Aromantic self.

In the twenty years that I've been treating patients with nature's essential oils I've seen some really remarkable transformations. Josie, for example, was a twenty-seven-year-old secretary in a law firm when she came to see me for back pain. Divorced and with no children, she was far too thin and was constantly depressed, irritable and snappy. I relieved the tension in her sacral region but the problem recurred – something was deeply wrong and eventually it came out: Josie had never had any pleasure from sex, absolutely no feeling at all. 'I've tried everything,' she told me, 'and I'd rather eat a packet of potato chips.' When I asked why she even bothered with sex, she replied forlornly, 'I don't want to be alone.'

We decided to try a new formula of bergamot, narcissus and jasmine. Slowly, Josie blossomed. Not only did the back pain completely disappear, but she began to put on weight and the colour returned to her face, which now looked quite different with a broad, bright smile. 'Now I know what it's all about,' she beamed. 'Sex is wonderful!'

Wonderful too are the essential oils. They each have their own character, which, as in people, is complex, subtle and sometimes paradoxical. You will find that there are oils which seem to be on the same wavelength as you, like good friends, and just as you will want to be with one friend but not another, so you will find yourself reaching for one oil and not another on a particular day. Preparing blends is like making a party list – some combinations work better than others. While some are for business, or health, others are just for outrageous fun.

Jasmine is what I call the 'empress' of oils. It is seductive and brings out the seductress in you! It seems to replace the element of femininity in a person, male or female, while at the same time relating to the person – rather as if one had had a soul-searching chat with a dear and helpful friend. It puts us back on course, refreshed. Ylang-ylang, on the other hand, is like an exotic friend from the Far East who is terribly intense but strangely relaxing and terrific in mixes (providing they aren't of the puritanical type!).

Clary-sage and fennel have female-hormone-like properties and are very helpful in dealing with sexual problems. You will often find them in my formulas to help menstrual problems and premenstrual tension, or in the formulas to overcome slow and prolonged arousal, the inability to have a sexual response or a general lack of libidinous desire.

But one doesn't have to have a problem to take advantage of the extraordinary benefits of essential oils. One can be the Aromantic woman any time. Start the day with an Aromantic bath or shower using, perhaps, an aroma to give yourself confidence, or one for going out and getting what you want! Perhaps you need an aroma to stimulate your general mood or one to keep you alert, aware of everything that's going on around. You will find here exclusive formulas to help overcome anxiety, stress and tension, sadness, fatigue, depression and feelings of insecurity. There are formulas to help if you are overworked; tonics for the nervous system; and cushions against the storm. Life is a hard struggle, but if your only problem is cellulite, the essential oils can help with that, too!

When you become an Aromantic woman you take advantage of the knowledge of ages and join the famous seductresses of history and legend. Circe, the original Greek enchantress, used nature's essential oils to keep Odysseus from his travels. According to legend, Helen of Troy acquired her fatal beauty from a formula given to her by Venus, the goddess of love. Cleopatra wasn't the great beauty Hollywood would have us believe, but a rather plain woman who used the essential oils to impress herself upon the hearts of Caesar, and then Mark Antony. With the purple sails of her royal barge soaked in rose water, Cleopatra's arrival was heralded by a sweet smell on the breeze long before her lovers could see the barge sailing towards them on the River Cydnus. She certainly knew how to make a lasting impression upon a man and was lucky enough to have the resources of an impressive civilization to help her out – it's said that she ordered a carpet of rose petals for Mark Antony's arrival. How much would such an extravagant gesture of romance cost you or I today, I wonder?

The Aromantic woman is getting back in harmony with nature and we are actually luckier than Cleopatra because we can tune in to precious oils from all over the world – thanks to sophisticated communication and transport facilities. Nature's rich treasury can be laid out before us in hundreds of little bottles containing the essential oils, a proportion of which come within the scope of this book. Cleopatra had to go to great lengths to ensure her supply of rose, frankincense and myrrh (which she put on her hair) and would have been jealous, I'm sure, if she knew of the subtle variety in nature's treasury available to us today.

Our knowledge has grown through the millennia with experience. The ancient Greek ladies would apply marjoram to the head, palm-oil to the face and essence of mint to the arms. The Book of Proverbs warned men long ago to beware of women who lured them to illicit beds perfumed with myrrh, cinnamon and oil of aloe. To the English, rosemary was the symbol of love and marriage and brides would adorn their veil with it. The little St John's Wort flower was included in silk or muslin sachets of love-herbs which girls wore next to their skin to attract the opposite sex. Chinese women wore the flower of the sambac tree in their heads or placed the petals in bowls around the house to allow the seductive, orange blossom-like aroma to delight the environment, their lovers, and themselves.

However, romance is not yet dead, and I'm reminded of an amusing incident told by my friend Susan. One night her boyfriend covered their bed with rose petals, but the petals squashed and stuck to them both like leeches. They spent half the night in the bathroom trying to wash them off! When I'd stopped laughing, I suggested to Susan that she keep some essential oils by the bed and put a few drops on the bedsheets before retiring – rose Maroc is heavy and passionate, Egyptian rose is seductive and persuasive, while rose Bulgar is romantic and sensual, and Turkish rose is gently erotic.

Making life a bed of roses is easy with the essential oils! Of course, Aromantics want petals, too. You can either add plain silk rose petals to the scene above, or make Aromantic rose petals – simply put the silk petals in a box, add a tissue or cottonwool pad with a couple of rose oil drops to the box, and shake and leave to set, as they say.

Silk absorbs the aroma of essential oils beautifully, and scattered on the pillows and sheets, Aromantic petals are a truly lovely alternative to the real thing. Sadly, as Susan also discovered, there is very little aroma left in the shop-bought rose – and is it any wonder when in all probability it's been overbred in a vast greenhouse and fed with chemical fertilizer?

Indeed, 'nature' is a different thing to what it used to be. Our ancestors walked through bean fields in bloom

113

in early summer, breathing in the scent which is said to cause a deep, positive, emotional reaction, while we walk through fluorescent-lit supermarkets to buy frozen beans in packets! When the advertising people say 'You've come a long way, baby', they're right – we've come a long way away from nature.

With the rich variety of oils and formulas, used in the many different ways, it's just a matter of experimenting until you find the oils and methods of use that work best for you. The Aromantic woman is aware of her moods and feelings because they are her guide to the oils most sympathetic to her at any given time. Above all, the Aromantic woman is positive, because essential oils are about enhancing the positive – and fulfilling potential.

The Especially Feminine Oils

Angelica ◆ Benzoin ◆ Bergamot ◆ Chamomile Roman
Clary-sage ◆ Coriander ◆ Cypress ◆ Fennel
Geranium ◆ Grapefruit ◆ Hyacinth ◆ Jasmine
Jonquil ◆ Lavender ◆ Lime ◆ Mandarine ◆ Marjoram
Neroli ◆ Nutmeg ◆ Patchouli ◆ Pettigraine ◆ Pimento
berry ◆ Rose Bulgar ◆ Rose Maroc ◆ Rosemary
Tonka bean ◆ Verbena ◆ Violet leaf ◆ Ylang-ylang

NEROLI is intensely female. It calms highly charged emotional states and redirects the energies. Relaxing yet stimulating, energetic and confident, it positively helps you to face emotional fear.

PATCHOULI has a masculine character and is earthy and profound. It stimulates the nervous system. For keeping awake – not for sleeping. Strident and forceful.

YLANG-YLANG is intensely sweet. Soothes away the frustrations of life. Excitingly exotic. Stimulates the senses. Dispels jealousy.

CLARY-SAGE is like a seductive man – it makes you heady and euphoric. But it's also profound. Calming away melancholy, stress and paranoia. Stimulates the sexual woman in you.

GRAPEFRUIT is a liquid face-lift. It brightens up the day or night – like a ray of sunshine warming your back and face. A booster oil full of positivity and confidence.

ROSE MAROC is luxurious, earthy yet erotically sexual. It's warm, dark and mysterious. If you use it you had better mean it! Good for confidence and bringing out your deepest feelings.

ANGELICA gets called in when the going gets tough. It will get you through. It won't solve your problems for you but it will help you see them in a new light. Changes sluggishness into revitalization.

JASMINE is powerful. Provokes the ultimate image of woman in a man. Seductive – it gently lifts your darkest moods. Flows through your anxieties, sedating and relaxing you.

PIMENTO BERRY is spicy and hot. Full-blooded suggestiveness. Physically passionate. Vivid and wild. Good for carnival time!

BENZOIN is warming and energizing. It's like wrapping up against the storm, or like eating chocolate. It penetrates the emotional shield and can provoke erotic thoughts.

BERGAMOT is original and persuasive. It coaxes you out of depression and enlivens your sexlife. It blanks out crises and allows you to get what you want.

NUTMEG is volatile and warm. It is desirability and availability! Provocative and seductive but calming and lingering. It disperses disturbing anxieties.

GERANIUM is friendly, sweet and kind. It balances the aggressive and passive effects of life. It creates harmony and good humour between the sexes, and irons out irrationality and discontent.

ROSE BULGAR gives emotional comfort and cossets you from the storm. It's sensuously feminine. Like wearing silk next to the skin. A confidence booster, like having a secret admirer. It enlivens your heart.

TONKA BEAN has exquisite intimacy. It links the deeper emotions in relationships, creating a euphoric cushion around events.

JONQUIL will bring out your hidden desires. It transcends the conscious mind; it's hypnotic. It dissolves frustrations and low self-esteem.

PETTIGRAINE is delicate, yet strong. It's trustworthy and helpful when you've been betrayed. It calms the anger and restores faith in yourself. It can positively strengthen.

HYACINTH is sweet and gentle – like a wood of bluebells in spring. It opens your heart and mind. Gives courage. Narcotic. It helps you to reach deep within yourself, so you blossom and bloom.

LAVENDER has a steadying influence on the psyche. Calming, yet intuitive, like a wise woman. Indecisiveness and emotional conflict are washed fresh away.

CORIANDER is uplifting and encouraging. It gently stimulates you into action. Spicy, warm and provocative.

LIME is intensely bittersweet. Can get you into action, but never discreetly! Think loud and egotistical – subtlety is not where lime is at!

VIOLET LEAF is mysterious and melancholy. It goes where no mortals dare. Silent, seductive and persuasive. Helps you to realize your potential.

CYPRESS is proud and enigmatic. It eases the sadness, yet is direct and outspoken. Helps you to stand up for yourself.

MANDARINE is young and fresh. Very sympathetic. Subtly inspiring and strengthening.

FENNEL helps a woman like a workout at the gym or a visit to the Well Woman clinic. It comforts and enlivens the personality.

MELISSA casts a spell of happiness. It's gentle and soft. It fizzes like sherbet – for the mentally exhausted and the lethargic it has a compelling potency.

CHAMOMILE ROMAN is golden. It humbly dispels nervousness and anger. Creates emotional stability – nothing can worry you now. It majestically clears away past emotional debris.

MARJORAM redirects the sexual energy, carrying away fear of love. Soothes the brokenhearted – when you need a cuddle and not sex. Warms the emotional cold.

ROSEMARY is royal in stature. It stimulates your sensitivity like ambrosia – the liquid of the gods. It increases creativity by lifting exhaustion and it philosophically awakens your heart.

THE AROMANTIC WOMAN *APRÈS L'AMOUR*

Après l'amour is a special time. When are we ever more relaxed? Lying close, soaking in the happy sensations together, touching gently, at peace with the world. *Après l'amour* is a time of giving thanks, and affirmation.

According to the ancient Chinese Taoist tradition, *après l'amour* is an especially alchemical time if the penis is allowed to rest in, or close to, the vagina after lovemaking. A wonderful exchange of male–female energies is said to take place as the chemicals in the sexual fluids are absorbed through the mucous membranes. To jump out of bed immediately after lovemaking to wash, for example, would be considered very bad form by the Chinese sages, because you would be denying your partner, as well as yourself, the medicinal benefits this intimate chemical exchange provides.

But whatever your tradition, *après l'amour* is no time to go rushing about. And why do so when you can have Aromantics at the flick of a switch? Simply reach out from under the bedclothes, turn on the bedside lamp and wait. As the lightbulb heats, so too will the few drops of essential oil you put on to it earlier, releasing the aroma into the atmosphere of the room. Just two or three drops will be enough to change your night.

Après l'amour is a mellow time, so make sure the lightbulb has a low wattage or, if you can find one, a love-rose hue. You don't want to break the special bond created between you by blinding your lover as you flick on an unshaded 100 watt bulb! Alternatively, put two or three drops of your chosen essential oil (or synergistic concentrate of oil) on to a cottonwool ball and pop it on to a radiator, or similar heat-source when, as they say, required.

Après l'amour massage is low key. With smooth, gentle movements, stroke your lover's forehead from the eyebrows to hairline, wishing his worries away. If you are prepared for more lovemaking, try a gentle massage of the erectile area of his lower back – a band about four inches high, just lower than his waist, at the centre by his vertebrae. Massage here, using one of the male stimulant oils that follow, will revive any man's interest in love.

Après l'amour is a sensitive time for many. The French have a saying: '*Après l'amour, les animaux sont toujours triste*' – after love, the animals are always sad. This is the observation, more often than not, of the swing between over-excitement and low melancholy, and something is needed to stop this swing and balance out the emotions. While some people find that talking after love is easy, others experience a silence which sharply echoes what is being left unsaid. To open channels of communication, try jonquil, but be warned – she reveals all. Clary-sage, on the other hand, is an opening and awakening oil.

Essential Oils for:

Balancing out emotions	Communication/ opening out	Accentuating the romantic	Accentuating the erotic
Geranium	*Jonquil*	*Palma rosa*	*Jasmine*
Bergamot	*Clary-sage*	*Hyacinth*	*Ylang-ylang*

Or maybe you want something to make *après l'amour* into 'more *amour*'? Because the aroma of the oils that stimulate your man into more amour don't appeal immediately to everyone, you can just as effectively mix them with an oil which accentuates the erotic – to his taste, and yours. Use a total of three drops on a heat-source or make a massage oil with these same 2:1 proportions – put twenty drops of a stimulating oil plus ten of a mixer into a 30 ml size bottle of pure vegetable or nut oil.

Stimulating Oils for Men		*Mixers*
Cumin	◄ *Use alone or*	*Ylang-ylang*
Costus	*blend 2 parts to 1*	*Palma rosa*
Cardamom	*part mixer* ►	*Jasmine*
Ambrette		*Carnation*
Anise		*Turkish rose*

And if you decide that you want a break from laidback *après l'amour* and yearn for some *après l'amour* zip, try grapefruit for physical and mental stimulation or lemon for a physically stimulating but mentally sedating effect. For those who like *l'amour* in the morning, a couple of drops of grapefruit on a face-cloth in the shower, or in the bath water, will put the best of the zest into your day.

Après l'amour is, above all, a time to harmonize. You are unique, your relationship is unique. Find for yourselves a blend uniquely right for you . . . *après l'amour*.

SENSUALITY AND CONFIDENCE

Sensuality and confidence are a reinforcing pair that go through life hand in hand. Without confidence, sensuality is lost. In this challenging world there are innumerable opportunities for confidence to be worn thin, so we need to build ourselves up.

In this section I shall be giving you my formulas to deal with a variety of things which affect a woman's confidence in herself. You may need a formula to help you go for it in the work world, or something to help you put yourself back together after a relationship break-up. You will find something here for depression, sadness, anxiety, stress, tension, and nerves that feel as though they've been through the shredder. But like the cavalry, the essential oils come to the rescue. Recover your inner confidence and your natural sensuality will bloom. So let's begin by looking at the oils best suited for generally raising confidence.

Confidence Boosters

Carnation	Tonka bean	Rosemary
Rose Bulgar	Vanilla	Grapefruit
Rose Maroc	Bergamot	Mace
Basil	Geranium	Nutmeg
Marjoram	Melissa	Neroli

Many of the essences mentioned here are highly sensual. Vanilla and tonka bean, for example, have a deep and profound odour which affects the emotions strongly, releasing pent-up angers and frustrations yet leaving you feeling calm. Bergamot, on the other hand, is a go-ahead, strident oil which banishes depressive moods. Quite a useful oil in this day and age! Grapefruit, again, has a different effect – it enlightens your heart, uplifting and stimulating.

Here are two terrific formulas for going out and getting what you want. Mix your synergistic concentrate as directed, then use it by putting three drops in the bath, or on a tissue for use when needed during the day.

Go for it Synergistic Blend No.1		Go for it Synergistic Blend No.2	
Tonka bean	4 drops	Rose Maroc	3 drops
Neroli	3 drops	Nutmeg	3 drops
Mace	3 drops	Bergamot	2 drops
Grapefruit	2 drops	Vanilla	4 drops

For those of you who need to be alert yet still aware of everything going on about you – a traffic cop, for example – a simple but very effective addition to your day could be basil or rosemary.

Next, we come to the essential oils that stimulate your general mood and help you to project yourself. In this group are oils that have a stimulatory effect on the adrenal cortex and give you a helping hand to alleviate stress. Clearly, a worried and stressed person cannot feel confidence or inspire much confidence in those around her. You can use the oils for stimulating your general mood on their own, but you might not find their perfume very attractive, so mix them with an antidepressant in a ratio of 2:1.

Oils for Stimulating your General Mood		Mixers (Antidepressants)
Rosemary	◄ Use oils alone, or	Bergamot
Basil	blend 1 part to 2	Lemon
Pine	parts 'mixer' ►	Orange
Thyme		Grapefruit
Savory		Lime

This last mixer, lime, is a great morale booster, giving us the zest that we took from the rind of the fruit in the first place. Nothing puts the zip into your day faster than a drop or two used on your face-cloth under the shower in the morning. If you're feeling as flat as a pancake because you've just broken up with your lover, lime can help. Lime and a night out with the girls is an excellent remedy; or try my Lost Love formula.

Lost Love Pick-You-Up

Lime	3 drops
Tonka bean	1 drop
Rose Maroc	1 drop

There are innumerable causes of sadness, which are often quite inexplicable, even to ourselves. Sadness often brings with it a feeling of dejection which gives off a silent signal. We usually know when someone is down. Bringing back a sense of happiness is not always possible with the essential oils, but if we cannot always make the sadness go away, the oils can bring enormous help, as they cushion us from the effects of life's many disappointments.

One such oil is rose Bulgar. Its effects on the emotions of women is unique, as hundreds of my patients can testify. Rose Bulgar gives a satisfaction and fulfilment in moments of crisis which people find difficult to explain. Its gentle aroma wraps itself around our innermost anxieties and sadnesses. Its fragrance is exquisite, although this in itself doesn't explain why its effect is primarily on women. Despite the fact that it is one of the most expensive essential oils in the world, a drop of rose Bulgar will cost you less than a drink to drown your sorrows and will be immeasurably more supportive and infinitely better for you.

Here is a formula to help you in your most difficult moments. Use three drops of the concentrate in the bath or one drop on a tissue or handkerchief, and breathe in when needed. I find that just two drops in a room diffuser works wonders for my psyche.

Cushion-Against-the-Storm
Synergistic Concentrate

Rose Bulgar	*4 drops*
Chamomile Roman	*1 drop*
Neroli	*2 drops*

Anxiety, stress and tension are so much a part of modern living that we hardly bat an eye when people fall seriously ill and the doctor says it's 'stress'. The illnesses are the result of 'a force acting on or within a thing and tending to distort it' – the dictionary definition of stress. Stress distorts us!

Sex is usually the first thing to suffer – it's difficult to be a vibrant, positive sexual being when we are actually exhausted by the negative vicissitudes of life. Luckily, nature has provided us with a rich store of helpmates.

The Woman's Helpmates for the Nervous System

Tonics	Both tonic and sedative	Sedatives
Cypress		Neroli
Marjoram	Geranium	Lemon
Rosemary	Marjoram	Marjoram
Tangerine	Lavender	Jasmine
Angelica	Neroli	Rose Maroc
Melissa	Tangerine	Bois de rose
Borage seed	Hyssop	Chamomile Roman
Hyssop	Bay	Nutmeg
Orange		Jonquil

Stress	Anxiety	Nervous depression	Tension
Rose Maroc	Rose Bulgar	Benzoin	Rose Maroc
Lemon	Bergamot	Chamomile Roman	Chamomile Roman
Jasmine	Ginger	Lavender	Nutmeg
Fennel	Lavender	Bergamot	Lavender
Hyssop	Orange	Thyme	Basil
Neroli	Melissa	Grapefruit	Jonquil
Geranium	Mandarine	Ylang-ylang	Coriander
Sandalwood	Marjoram	Jasmine	Rosemary
			Rose Bulgar

The best way to use women's helpmate oils, alone or in a synergistic concentrate, is in a bath, in a massage oil, in a room diffuser, or simply wear the oil as a perfume.

Some days are just hectic. When I'm overworked, overtired, rushed off my feet and my muscles are aching, there's nothing better than a good long soak in my rescue formula bath.

The Rescue Formula

Grapefruit	3 drops
Ginger	2 drops
Ylang-ylang	1 drop

We all encounter stress and tension and here are some formulas for baths to revive you. Some people prefer showers and find the whole idea of bathing – washing in your own dirt, so to speak – distasteful. If that is so, then simply shower beforehand to get rid of the dirt and then have your stress-relieving bath!

Five Baths to Relieve Stress and Tension

Lemon	3 drops	Geranium	3 drops	Lavender	3 drops
Coriander	2 drops ◇	Mandarine	2 drops ◇	Basil	1 drop
Nutmeg	1 drop	Rosemary	1 drop	Lemon	2 drops

Bergamot	2 drops	Neroli	4 drops
Rose Maroc	3 drops ◇	Jasmine	3 drops
Nutmeg	1 drop	Chamomile Roman	1 drop

There are some women who suffer stress because they have a worry which is troubling them and making them feel uneasy. If this includes you, try my bath formula to lessen anxiety.

The Anti-Anxiety
Bath Formula

Sandalwood	3 drops
Jonquil	1 drop
Bergamot	2 drops

If you have a kind, loving partner on hand, one of the most effective ways to combat stress and tension is to luxuriate in an Aromantic massage. Massage is wonderful for stress and tension at any time. Choose one of the formulas below, added to 30 ml of vegetable oil. They will transform your battle-weary form into a positively confident Aromantic woman.

Three Body Massage Oils for Stress and Tension

Neroli	8 drops	Tangerine	8 drops	Lavender	10 drops
Geranium	7 drops ◇	Rosemary	5 drops ◇	Chamomile Roman	2 drops
Coriander	4 drops	Jonquil	2 drops	Bergamot	3 drops

Here is one of my all-time favourite formulas. All the oils come from the orange tree – pettigraine from the twigs, neroli from the flowers and orange from the fruit – and this reunited whole gives us a roundness, a wholeness, too. The formula seems to penetrate every part of our being, while the scent uplifts.

Reuniting the Whole Formula

Pettigraine	2 drops
Neroli	3 drops
Orange	1 drop

Add this formula to the bath, or make a concentrate and use one or two drops to perfume the room.

◇

Reuniting the Whole Body Massage Formula

Pettigraine	4 drops
Neroli	8 drops
Orange	3 drops

In 30 ml of vegetable oil

Loving, and being loved in return is, of course, the biggest confidence booster. The essential oils of nature give you their love, strange as that may seem. Their love is not judgemental, but sympathetic and helpful. They help you fulfil your potential as a vibrant human being and to this end will support you in many different ways. If you love yourself enough to allow the oils to give you their special love, then even more love will be attracted to you – the Aromantic woman.

LOW SEXUAL RESPONSE

Low is a word about relativity: low is simply lower than higher. It could be that you just want to increase your desire and libido. Or perhaps you are unable to contemplate intercourse at all. No matter, there is something in Aromantics for everyone.

The Sexy Oils

Anis vert	Jasmine	Ginger
Clove	Cinnamon	Hyssop
Clary-sage	Fenugreek	Juniper
Mace	Fennel	Peppermint
Pine	Neroli	Rosemary
Sage	Rose Maroc	Sandalwood
Thyme	Savory	Angelica
Mint	Ylang-ylang	Ambrette
	Cumin	

There is nothing new about utilizing components of nature's store house to increase libido. Sixteen centuries ago the *Kama Sutra* suggested readers try mimosa, cassia, myrtle and myrrh to excite desire, and the call for aphrodisiacs continues to this day.

We start with formulas to increase desire. There are two, as good as each other, so choose the one whose aroma appeals most to you.

Blends to Increase Desire

Floral massage formula			Spicy massage formula	
Jasmine	6 drops	◀ *Each formula* ▶	Cinnamon	3 drops
Rose Maroc	6 drops	*in 30 ml of*	Mace	4 drops
Sandalwood	10 drops	*vegetable oil*	Nutmeg	4 drops
Cumin	8 drops		Coriander	3 drops
			Tonka bean	5 drops
			Ylang-ylang	10 drops

Floral bath formula			Spicy bath formula	
Jasmine	1 drop	◀ *On the* ▶	Nutmeg	2 drops
Rose Maroc	2 drops	*bath*	Coriander	1 drop
Sandalwood	2 drops	*water*	Ylang-ylang	1 drop
Cumin	1 drop			

Next, we have the sexy formulas. Try the one that seems to reflect you best at this particular time, and like any menu, you can pick and choose different options on different days. Try them all! I'm sure there's a formula included here which will lift your sex life to new heights –just give the formula a chance to work. After two or three applications you should be feeling more responsive.

The Sexy Synergistic Blends

Over-tense

Rose Maroc	5 drops
Sweet fennel	2 drops
Sandalwood	2 drops

◇

Over-anxious and tense

Mace	2 drops
Anise	1 drop
Cinnamon	1 drop
Neroli	5 drops

◇

Insecure

Rose Maroc	6 drops
Clary-sage	2 drops
Clove	1 drop

Fatigued

Rosemary	3 drops
Neroli	3 drops
Cumin	3 drops

◇

Overworked

Anise	2 drops
Sandalwood	5 drops
Ginger	2 drops

Unable to have a sexual response

Angelica	3 drops
Clary-sage	4 drops
Sandalwood	2 drops

◇

Arousal is slow and prolonged

Rose Maroc	5 drops
Ylang-ylang	2 drops
Ginger	2 drops

◇

Sad

Angelica	3 drops
Rose Maroc	3 drops
Ylang-ylang	2 drops
Cumin	2 drops

Depressed

Rose Maroc	3 drops
Neroli	4 drops
Rosemary	2 drops

◇

Faraway and distant

Savory	1 drop
Ylang-ylang	4 drops
Ginger	2 drops
Clary-sage	9 drops

Sexual vibrancy is affected by many factors, often two or three at the same time which, in their conjunction, freeze the sexual psyche. Woman's sexual coldness is often attributed to some hypothetical physical inability but rarely, for example, to her man's emotional coldness. But we have to look at the whole in sex because while sex is many things, there is one thing it is not – simple! With nature's essential oils at hand, we have a very good chance of loosening the blocks to sexual vibrancy providing the woman actually wants to be vibrant with her man. This has to be said – the essential oils are pretty fantastic, but they won't miraculously transform a man you don't love into one that you do.

Another difficult block to sexual vibrancy is deep-seated sadness. Whatever its root cause – and the cause can be quite forgotten and subconscious – sadness often stays inside and hidden, something we are unable to release. We may instinctively realize, however, that to release the sadness would involve the release of emotional pain and it can seem simpler to suppress the whole problem as best we can. Unfortunately, the body isn't as good at suppression as it is at relocation and the block could simply get transferred to the sexual area.

This brings us to the 'Blockbuster' formulas. These are very good at bringing out the Aromantic in a woman who desires the warmth and companionship of a man but does not desire sexual intercourse. The oils have a cumulative effect, so just try, slowly but surely, to unloose the blocks by finding and using the oil or the formula best suited to you. As a general guide, use daily and expect to see subtle changes in seven to nine days. Make up a formula to your own aroma taste, as directed below.

Blockbuster Oils

Group A	Group B
Ylang-ylang	*Savory*
Jasmine	*Mace*
Clary-sage	*Cumin*
	Cinnamon
	Ginger

▲ | ▲

Use 10–20 drops maximum of any of these . . . | *Use up to 5 drops maximum of any of these . . .*

. . . to a total of 30 drops per 30 ml of vegetable oil

For baths, use a maximum of three drops of any one oil in group A plus a maximum of one drop of any one oil in group B. Alternatively, try one of my Blockbuster bath formulas.

Three Blockbuster Baths

Cinnamon	1 drop	Savory	1 drop	Jasmine	3 drops
Ylang-ylang	2 drops ◇	Ginger	2 drops ◇	Ginger	1 drop
Cumin	3 drops	Sage	1 drop	Mace	2 drops

Or try a Blockbuster massage oil formula.

Two Blockbuster Body Massage Oils

Savory	2 drops	◀ In 30 ml of ▶	Mace	5 drops
Ginger	5 drops	vegetable	Jasmine	10 drops
Cinnamon	3 drops	oil	Ginger	5 drops
Ylang-ylang	15 drops		Ylang-ylang	5 drops
			Cinnamon	5 drops

The human sexual experience is all about potential – we can have lows and highs. For years I have been watching lows turn into highs, ill health turn into radiant good health, as my patients confidently blossom in the light of the essential oils of nature. Their effect is truly remarkable. When I see such changes taking place it's clear to me that we were meant to be happy sexual beings because, in being fulfilled sexually, we're better able to face the many challenges of life with love, strength, humour and happiness. Moreover, a good sexual relationship is better able to withstand the strains put upon it by a life full of choices.

Humanity has always turned to nature for strength, but perhaps there has never been a time when nature has been so distanced from people and yet so needed. The essential oils are nature at its most concentrated and effective, so turn to nature, become the Aromantic woman and rejoice!

DOUCHES

When you use a douche, you're putting foreign substances right on to some of the most delicate membranes
in your entire body. It is very important to realize two
things. First, the volumes I give in this section must be
strictly adhered to – there is absolutely no need to
exceed the recommended quantities of essential oil that
you add to your douche water – indeed, it can be
dangerous to do so. Don't say to yourself, 'I have a
greater need therefore I will use a greater quantity', say
instead, '. . . therefore I shall use the oils for a longer
period of time than someone else may need to.'

The second thing is that precisely because the
vagina's mucous membrane is of such a delicate,
absorbent nature, the molecules of nature's essential
oils very quickly and effectively enter the body and do
their work. For some conditions, douches can be the
most successful method of treatment. But, please note,
*pregnant women should not douche with essential oils or any
other substances unless medically advised.*

Not every woman uses a douche – in America they
are in widespread use while in Britain they are not. This
difference has more to do with the fact that Americans
prefer showers while the British love nothing better
than a long soak with a rubber duck. Obviously, when
you lie in the bath the water enters you and gives you a
douche, so duck-lovers don't feel the need for special
douching equipment, as the Americans do. Some
British women will never have seen a douche in their
entire lives, although most chemists do stock them, and
to them I say that a douche is a rubber bag (which you
fill with water) with a nozzle attached. This is put into
the vagina to allow the water to enter and wash the
vagina out. In Europe there seems to be a balance –
women sometimes shower and sometimes bath – and
most European women own a douche. A British friend
of mine was made to feel like a naughty schoolgirl when
she told a French doctor that she didn't possess a
douche she could use for the medication he had given

her. In Japan, where bathing, even communal bathing, is a national tradition, douches were introduced from America and originally sold on the Tupperware home-party principle. As I understand it, one of the things that clinched sales was the idea that douching reduced the length of periods – a very doubtful point, but it certainly helped sales.

The use of douches in the treatment of vaginal infections is widespread and, if prescribed by your doctor, quite safe. However, researchers at America's National Institutes of Health are recommending that women use vinegar and water in their douches, rather than the commercial chemical preparations Americans have been using in recent years. The sales of these preparations have tripled in the past twelve years, a fact, the researchers think, not unrelated to the rise over the past ten years in the incidence of ectopic pregnancies among American women.

The danger in using chemical products (when 'strawberry' is more chemical flavouring than strawberry) is that they destroy the naturally protective organisms that live in the vagina. The researchers at NIH think that daily douching could slowly wear away the mucous plug in the cervical canal. Clearly, one has to take care and douche in moderation.

When using essential oils in douches it is absolutely *vital* to ensure that you are buying the pure product. If you intend to use douches, now is the time to make the effort to shop around to find the best essential oil supplier in town. Don't accept the assurance of sales staff that their oils are pure – they may simply not know the difference.

Having said that, you will be perfectly safe if you follow the four golden rules for making an Aromantic douche:

1. *You cannot use every essential oil in a douche. Do not suppose that formulas given elsewhere in this book can also be used in douches. Some essential oils will burn the mucous membrane of the vagina. Never take the risk; only use the oils suggested in this*

134

section or those I have specifically suggested for use in douches in other sections.

2. *Never use more than eight drops of essential oil in each pint of water. This is a ratio of one drop to 2 fl oz. Bear that in mind, and always follow the 1:2 rule. If your douche is not size-marked, fill it and then empty the water into a measuring jug so that you know the capacity once and for all.*

3. *Always dilute the essential oil in pure spring water that has been boiled. Then filter the mixture through a paper coffee filter and leave to cool to body temperature. Don't use the water too hot or too cold as this can be harmful to the mucous membrane of the vagina.*

4. *Douche a maximum of twice a week, and then for the limited period of time as directed.*

In this section we shall be discussing the essential oils that are for cleansing and purifying, as well as those for increasing sexual response. So, to start, pour into a measuring jug 1 pint/560 ml of cooled boiled water and add your chosen essential oil. The essential oils and water do not mix – some, like lavender, will spread across the surface of the water while others, like benzoin, may drop to the bottom. Mix as best you can and if your jug has a detachable top, shake the jug, and filter the mixture through a paper coffee filter. Pour the solution into the douche bag and use in the normal way, according to the type of equipment you have.

Vinegar-and-water douches have been popular for a very long time, but don't think the proportions are meant to be 50:50. If you see vinegar-and-water being recommended somewhere, bear in mind that you should never add more than 20 per cent vinegar to 80 per cent water. Vinegar is a good addition to a douche, however, in small quantities, because it maintains the acidity of the vagina. Here is my preferred method: mix together 5 ml (one teaspoon) of cider vinegar with 1 ml (or twenty drops) of your chosen essential oil or synergistic blend. When you want to make a douche add two drops of this mixture to every one fluid ounce of water. In other words, if your douche holds one pint/

560 ml add thirty-two drops of your pre-prepared vinegar–oil mixture to boiled, cooled water and filter. You can prepare several solutions for different purposes and keep them on hand, ready for use.

If you don't have a douche there are other methods you can use, although they aren't as effective. On the continent, women use bidets for their vaginal baths. If you don't have a bidet, simply lower yourself into a bowl of lukewarm water into which you have put two to three drops of your chosen essential oil or synergistic blend of oils which have been previously diluted in one teaspoon of vegetable oil. In both cases, direct the water into your vagina by holding the entrance open with one hand and moving your other hand under the water, encouraging the water inside the vagina. Do this for as long as it takes for the water to circulate in and out several times.

Another variation on this theme, quite common in Europe, is called a 'sitz bath' and simply means that you fill a bath to the level of your hips, add up to five drops of essential oil which have been previously diluted in one teaspoon of vegetable oil – and sitz! Agitate the water in the same way, directing it into your vagina. The sitz bath, bidet and bowl methods have quite good results for the treatment of low sexual response.

Cleansing and purifying

For too long now women have been brainwashed into thinking that their vaginas smell. In my practice I see the result – women who live in constant fear that everyone can smell their intimate sexual aroma. In continental Europe the attitude is less paranoid and more practical. Women don't douche to wash away their own sexual aroma so much as to get rid of semen – *male* sexual aroma. Men smell too!

The fact of the matter is that anyone – male or female – will smell in the genital area if they don't wash away the dead bacteria that accumulate, either around the vulva or under the foreskin. And yet you never see commercial deodorant products for the penis or scrotum – the implication being that men don't smell, while women do. We need to distinguish between healthy, natural aroma, and smells which indicate that something is wrong. Simply squishing up our noses and spraying all manner of chemical products into ourselves is to ignore the signals our life-saving nose detects.

Reading the adverts you could be easily led to believe that smelling like a strawberry milkshake is preferable to smelling like your natural self. But nature put the apocrine glands into our genital area so that we would produce pheromones and attract the opposite sex. Ask yourself, who are we to trust – nature or the advertisers who make money by encouraging genital paranoia? I mean, do you want to attract another strawberry milkshake or do you want a real-life, sexy man?

Nature's oils operate on a completely different level to chemical suppressants. When you use essential oils you are adding more pheromones, albeit sweet-smelling plant ones, to your own. Men will find you doubly attractive!

Beside the 'birds and bees' connotations, essential oils have other advantages – they cleanse thoroughly and gently, have antibiotic, disinfectant and, in some cases, antifungal and antiviral properties. These oils do their job and they smell gorgeous while they do it. What more can one ask for?

Cleansing and Purifying Essential Douche Oils

Rose Bulgar	Clary-sage	Mandarine
Rose Maroc	Geranium	Calendula
Turkish rose	Tea tree	Cedarwood
Lavender	Ylang-ylang	Cypress
Rosemary	Bergamot	Lemon
Fennel	Neroli	Lime
Thyme	Marjoram	Jasmine
	Orange	

Use any one or any two, to a total of 2 drops to 1 pint/560 ml of water

When deciding which oil, or two oils, to use for cleansing and purifying, you could match the aroma to your bath oil or perfume. Alternatively, you could choose an oil that also serves another purpose. For example, if you need something to boost your confidence, douche with neroli.

Any of the rose oils are excellent for cleansing and purifying the female reproductive system. Rose is, in fact, known as the 'female-problem oil', because of its great usefulness in treating women. As if that weren't enough, rose is a marvellous relaxant, it's good for all skin complaints (including the wrinkles of age) and smells absolutely fabulous. No cosmetic or perfume manufacturer could do without rose and no woman should be without this most wonderful aid. A douche of rose once a week leaves you feeling fresh, alive and full of confidence – a strange thing for a douche to do, but it really does! Remember, the essential oils affect many levels, both physical and emotional.

As a matter of interest, the discovery of *attar* of rose, essence of rose, has been credited to the Indian empress, Nur Jehan Begum, in 1612, although it was known of long before this. The story goes that as she walked with the emperor beside the rose-water canal, bordered by flowers in the palace garden, Nur Jehan noticed a light, semi-solid foam floating along on top of the running canal water. She collected this 'foam' – concentrated rose essence – and her use of it no doubt contributed, along with her ingenuity, to her becoming the Sultan's favourite wife.

Any of the flower oils are going to smell good. Lavender is especially fresh and enlivening, while jasmine has the most marvellous seductive aroma and is renowned the world over as an aphrodisiac.

Depending on your own Aromantic taste, choose a fruity douche from orange, lemon or mandarine. You may prefer the herbal oils – rosemary, fennel, thyme or marjoram – which you can use on their own or mix with one of the other essential oils.

By mixing any two essential oils on the 'Cleansing

and purifying' list, or using any one of the oils alone, there are about two hundred permutations to choose from. From the choice you can identify the oil or combination of oils that suits you beautifully and, providing your oils are absolutely pure, you can be sure that your Aromantic douche will be doing you infinitely more good than any shop-bought mixture. Unlike some chemical preparations, Aromantic douches don't stop the vaginal secretions or leave a feeling of dryness. Instead, they leave you feeling pure and clean and quite delicious!

Low sexual response

Many women who had never experienced orgasm did so after a few weeks of using an Aromantic douche – but one doesn't have to have a problem . . . we can all go higher!

One of the marvellous things about sex is that it's a never ending adventure, full of new experiences. Certainly, with the potential for subtle variation, there should be no reason whatsoever for any loving couple to get bored. Life outside the bedroom provides quite enough material for a dynamic element to be brought into our intimate relationships. Unless we have a really boring relationship and a flat, dull sex life, new facets of the experience should be revealing themselves with subtlety continuously throughout our lives.

Essential Douche Oils to Increase Sexual Response

Aniseed	Rose Maroc	Sandalwood
Fennel	Ylang-ylang	Narcissus
Rosemary	Patchouli	Cardamom
Clary-sage	Ginger (but never more than 1 drop per pint)	Jasmine

Use any one or two, to a total of 2 drops to 1 pint/560 ml of water

139

If lovemaking seems likely on a particular night, use the essential oils to increase sexual response in the morning or the early evening. Jasmine is a great relaxant and cleanser with aphrodisiac qualities, especially good for women who have a tendency towards nervousness. Ylang-ylang has much the same effect. If you have what I call 'sexual debility' – you're feeling sexually weak and feeble because you're tense and mentally exhausted – try a douche of clary-sage or geranium.

Here, then, is a formula for everyone, whether or not you are experiencing low sexual arousal. Many of my clients who were already quite happy with their sexuality have tried this formula to enhance their sexual feeling – with exciting results. This is the formula that proves that the Aromantic way is the way up!

The Super-Sexy Synergistic Blend Douche

Jasmine	1 drop	*Make up a synergistic blend*
Rose Maroc	2 drops	*using these proportions,*
Sandalwood	2 drops	*then use 3 drops per pint/560 ml*
Ylang-ylang	2 drops	*of water (or water-vinegar mix)*

Now we come to the more specialized sexy douche formulas. All these are designed to heighten your sexual experience, so choose the one that seems to be most appropriate for you at this particular time. Again, these are synergistic blends, although the dose is different from the 'super-sexy' douche above. In these below, use one drop of the blend to every two fluid ounces of boiled, cooled water.

You're a nervous panicky type		You're overanxious and tense		You need to relax	
Jasmine	4 drops	Narcissus	3 drops	Rosemary	4 drops
Ylang-ylang	3 drops ◇	Clary-sage	5 drops ◇	Rose Maroc	5 drops
Clary-sage	2 drops	Jasmine	7 drops	Cardamom	2 drops
Rose Bulgar	7 drops	Ginger	1 drop	Patchouli	3 drops

You're disinterested in sex		Your arousal is too slow		Your arousal is too quick	
Jasmine	7 drops	Cardamom	5 drops	Narcissus	4 drops
Ylang-ylang	4 drops ◇	Sandalwood	2 drops ◇	Jasmine	7 drops
Clary-sage	3 drops	Rosemary	7 drops	Ylang-ylang	3 drops
		Rose Maroc	9 drops		
		Fennel	5 drops		

By all means, experiment with the oils; but so long as you *only* use the oils I have recommended in this section, and as long as you're sure that the essential oils you are using are absolutely pure, a weekly douche can give new meaning to the expression 'onwards and upwards'!

THE CYCLE OF LIFE

Whether we actually have children or not, the woman's body was designed for childbearing and is consequently highly intricate and sensitive. It is likely that at some time in our lives we will encounter one or other of the infections and problems that seem to be woman's lot. It's very difficult, however, to be the Aromantic woman if you're suffering real pain or discomfort. It can take all the energy you have simply to get through the day, with the night becoming a time to sleep, forget and gather enough strength to get through another prob-lematic day.

Sexual energy is the life energy directed towards the sexual area, and if your energy is being directed towards dealing with your gynaecological problem, there's not going to be much energy left over for sex. There is no avoiding the fact that your physical well-being is vital for your sexual well-being, your sexual relationship, your family relationships and your working life. So let's try to get your vehicle through life, your body, into good working order so that you can continue your journey in comfort and tranquillity – the sensuous Aromantic woman.

Premenstrual tension

I've known many women who, on their own admission, turn into 'monsters' the week before their period is due. Symptoms can range from a complete change of personality and character, comfort eating, constipation, nausea, acne, herpes attacks, backache, weight gain and water retention, to headaches, migraine, swollen abdomen, tender breasts, irrationality, loss of confidence, loss of libido, aggression, anger and so on. Any one of these symptoms can suffocate romance.

Some of the premenstrual stories I've heard from patients would be funny if they weren't also very frightening. Otherwise perfectly balanced women go around the house screaming, or they kick the children, the dog, the cat or the car, they throw plants and other handy projectiles at the poor confused lover and break down in floods of tears when they see their huge bloated stomach in the mirror!

A finely tuned hormonal balance is crucial to a woman's well-being, and premenstrual tension occurs when a woman becomes oversensitive to her own sexual hormones. What we need are nature's essential oils, in all their glorious peace, to counterbalance the condition.

Treatment must be started on the last day of menstruation and continued throughout the cycle, including the next menstruation. It could take two or three months before the cycle has settled down completely, but for sufferers, I can promise, the results are well worth waiting for.

An important part of the treatment of all menstrual-related problems is the base-oil with which you mix the essential oils. Unfortunately, the best oils are also the most expensive but you'll be able to afford them because you'll be saving money elsewhere – on buying replacement plants, for example! Bear in mind that some of these base-oils are as therapeutic as the essential oils themselves, so do try to use them.

The best base-oils are hazelnut, grapeseed and apricot kernel, to which a percentage of an oil that stimulates the production of prostaglandins, the active substance that helps premenstrual tension, should be added. Scientific tests have shown that borage seed oil contains twice as much essential fatty acids and gamma-linoleic acid (GLA) as evening primrose oil, and GLA helps to produce prostaglandins. Use borage seed oil if possible. (It can help too if you also take borage seed or evening primrose capsules alongside this essential oil treatment.)

When you massage yourself, rub the oil into your abdomen, over the hips and over the lower back to the coccyx – the lower end of the backbone, between the cleavage of the buttocks but not as far as the anus. But first, we have to prepare our massage oil.

30 ml base-oil – one of these:	Plus ▶	30 drops GLA oil additive – one of these:	Plus ▶	30 drops essential oil –
Hazelnut oil		*Borage seed oil*		*Single or*
Grapeseed oil		*Evening primrose oil*		*mixture chosen*
Apricot kernel oil				*from list below*

PMT Massage Oils

Bergamot	Jasmine	Galbanum
Rose Bulgar	Jonquil	Anise
Lavender	Mandarine	Sage
Geranium	Cypress	Rosemary
Clary-sage	Savory	Cardamom

I have found that the following combinations work well and you may like to try one of them.

Five PMT Body Massage Formulas

Rose Maroc	10 drops	Clary-sage	10 drops	Rosemary	10 drops
Geranium	10 drops ◇	Mandarine	10 drops ◇	Lavender	10 drops
Bergamot	10 drops	Cypress	10 drops	Geranium	10 drops

Cardamom	15 drops		Jonquil	5 drops
Jasmine	10 drops	◇	Bergamot	10 drops
Bergamot	5 drops		Cypress	15 drops

Massage daily, starting on the last day of menstruation and continue thereafter – as I have said, it could take two or three months before the cycle settles down. To this regime you should add a daily essential bath for seven days before your next menstruation is due. Add seven drops, chosen from the following oils, either singly or in a combination.

PMT Bath Oils

Geranium	Benzoin
Rose Bulgar	Tonka bean
Hyacinth	Bergamot
Narcissus	Chamomile Roman
Jonquil	Grapefruit

Alternatively, try one of the formulas suggested below.

Five PMT Bath Formulas

Bergamot	3 drops		Hyacinth	3 drops		Tonka bean	3 drops
Geranium	3 drops	◇	Chamomile		◇	Grapefruit	3 drops
			Roman	3 drops			

Rose Bulgar	4 drops		Narcissus	3 drops
Bergamot	2 drops	◇	Bergamot	3 drops

Menstrual problems

The most common menstrual problem is dysmenor-rhoea – painful periods. Providing there are no physical complications this problem can be helped by aromatherapy treatment or, indeed, at home.

Oils to Help Painful Periods

Anis vert	Cypress	Rosemary
Cajeput	Estragen	Sage
Chamomile Roman	Juniper	Nutmeg
	Peppermint	

Disregard old wives' tales about not bathing while you are having your period. Your best remedy is to have a daily essential oil bath in conjunction with a daily massage, which helps eliminate congestion, for a week beginning on the first day of your period. For the bath, choose any single or combination of essential oils from the list above – up to a total of five drops.

Apply your massage oil on the first day of your period, massaging over the whole of your abdomen and lower back and hips. Spend at least one minute doing this – although this doesn't sound like a long time, in practice it can seem so. Make up your massage oil for painful periods following the instructions below.

27 ml base-oil (90 per cent) – Plus ▶ one of these:	3 ml GLA oil (10 per cent) Plus ▶ – one of these:	30 drops per 30 ml *of any single or combination of essential oils on above list*
Hazelnut oil Grapeseed oil Apricot kernel oil	Borage seed oil Evening primrose oil	

An easy way to measure is to figure that you need just under five and a half teaspoons (5.4) of base-oil (e.g. hazelnut) and just over half a teaspoon (0.6) of GLA oil (borage or evening primrose). To this, you add the thirty drops of essential oil. If you follow the millilitre volumes given here, you will have enough to fill a smallish egg cup, which will be enough to last you the week. Here are the formulas.

Three Body Massage Formulas for Painful Periods

Nutmeg	10 drops	Sage	10 drops	Cypress	10 drops
Rosemary	10 drops ◇	Peppermint	10 drops ◇	Estragen	10 drops
Chamomile Roman	10 drops	Cajeput	10 drops	Rosemary	10 drops

Despite the fact that periods are painful and a nuisance, when they don't arrive that can be even more of a problem! Lack of menstruation is called amenorrhoea, and unless it is the result of early menopause, it is a condition which should be checked by your doctor. It could indicate a structural defect or hormone imbalance. On the physical level, amenorrhoea is the result of ovulation not occurring and therefore the lining of the uterus is not shed.

If you have previously had periods and now do not, you're diagnosed as having 'secondary' amenorrhoea. Women who are pregnant or lactating have this but, of course, there's no problem – this is normal. Most usually, secondary amenorrhoea is the result of emotional factors – perhaps a change of home, dieting, anxiety or stress. Mary Queen of Scots had amenorrhoea for eighteen months and was convinced she was pregnant. Perhaps she had an inkling of her fate – enough to give anyone amenorrhoea.

For those of you whose periods are absent or irregular, use the oils below daily for two months as they can often bring back regularity.

Oils for Irregular Periods or Absence of Periods

Rose Bulgar	Chamomile Roman	Lavender
Rose Maroc	Cypress	Nutmeg
Geranium	Peppermint	Thyme
Sage	Fennel	

Use them in a daily massage, massaging over your lower abdomen and hips, down to the crease of your buttocks.

Those who have a complete absence of periods can, alternatively, try one of my formulas below, in 30 ml of vegetable or nut oil.

Three Body Massage Oil Formulas for Absence of Periods

Rose Maroc	8 drops	Sage	8 drops	Red thyme	8 drops
Cypress	8 drops ◇	Geranium	8 drops ◇	Chamomile	
Fennel	8 drops	Lavender	8 drops	Roman	8 drops
				Peppermint	8 drops

Bleeding is an integral part of womanhood, but there are times when bleeding is a sign of danger. Unless you have just lost your virginity, bleeding after intercourse should never be ignored. The same goes for bleeding after you've been through the menopause – get it checked right away.

Lack of vaginal secretion

The amount of vaginal secretion before and during intercourse can vary enormously – largely depending upon our degree of sexual excitement. The absence of vaginal secretion, aside from making penetration difficult and sometimes impossible, is very upsetting for the man, who can feel rejected.

The menopause can reduce vaginal secretion and, during this time, one of the best ways to overcome the problem is to continue making love and having orgasms! Other reasons for lack of vaginal secretion are fright, anxiety, stress and tension, and when discussing these we must always remember that the cause can often be subconscious – we just don't know why we 'dry up'. Because of this it would be wrong to automatically assume that lack of secretion is the result of not finding your partner attractive, although you must seriously ask yourself whether this is, in fact, the root cause of the problem.

Vaginal secretions vary in their amount and consistency at different times during the menstrual cycle. During sexual excitement the Bartholin's glands, which lie right behind the entrance to the vagina, secrete a liquid which enables the penis to enter. The precise mechanism of the internal vaginal secretion release during the female sexual response is, however, still something of a controversy, but clearly relates to hormonal and sexual excitement levels.

The use of nature's essential oils for whatever purpose seems to increase the amount of vaginal secretions. Many generations of patients and therapists alike have noted this change. Your condition could be overcome then, simply by using the oils for another reason. Some essential oils seem to increase the supply of vaginal secretion more than others, mainly those that imitate the oestrogen hormone. No special treatment is required for this condition – a simple bath or massage oil will do the trick. I've had great success in treating this condition, so take heart from the fact that other sufferers have overcome the problem and gone on to recover their sensuality.

Oils for Treating Lack of Vaginal Secretion

Geranium	Sandalwood	Hyacinth	Cinnamon
Rose Bulgar	Ylang-ylang	Lavender	Nutmeg
Clary-sage	Neroli	Savory	Benzoin
Melissa	Cypress	Anise	Fennel

You can make up your own massage formula using the oils above. Add 10 per cent of an oil that is cosmetically good for the skin (borage seed, jojoba, evening primrose or carrot) to 90 per cent ordinary vegetable oil. Add thirty drops of essential oil to this base mixture of oils, shake gently and apply as you would any body oil, paying special attention to the lower abdomen, breasts and small of the back.

Three Body Massage Oil Formulas to Overcome Lack of Vaginal Secretion

Geranium	10 drops	Sandalwood	15 drops	Cypress	5 drops
Lavender	10 drops ◇	Neroli	5 drops ◇	Hyacinth	10 drops
Fennel	10 drops	Melissa	4 drops	Clary-sage	15 drops

For baths, the essential oils can be used singly – rose Bulgar is pure indulgent luxury, and good for you too! – or in a mixture. Here is a really lovely formula for the synergistic blend.

The Synergistic Blend for Lack of Vaginal Secretion

Rose Bulgar		Mix together into
(or) Maroc	10 drops	a concentrate
Clary-sage	10 drops	then add 6 drops
Fennel	2 drops	to each bath
Hyacinth	2 drops	

Or use one of the following bath formulas.

149

Three Bath Formulas to Overcome Lack of Vaginal Secretion

Rose Bulgar	4 drops	Geranium	2 drops	Cypress	1 drop
Geranium	1 drop	◇ Lavender	2 drops ◇	Hyacinth	2 drops
Melissa	1 drop	Fennel	2 drops	Clary-sage	3 drops

There are endless variations you may try for yourself. Allow about a week of both daily baths and massage before increased secretion is obtained, although most women find that after the third day their vaginas have a nice healthy level of secretion, penetration is easier and any discomfort previously experienced by a dry vagina has gone. Before closing on this subject I must just say one thing. In my practice I see many women who suffer this problem, including some who have endometriosis, yet they and many others – perhaps including yourself – will endure pain because they think they owe 'conjugal rights' to their partner. I've often heard a woman say 'He's ever so good' if her partner doesn't demand his 'rights' seven nights a week! If you haven't yet been to your gynaecologist, please do so now, as pain during intercourse can mean something more serious. Also, talking the problem over with your man can often dispel the psychological problems you may both be suffering because of the situation.

FERTILITY

The tragedy of childlessness is growing. In both the UK and USA, about one couple in six who attempt to conceive a child, fail. A study, by the American National Center for Health Statistics, of married women in the 20–24 age group – normally the most fertile – discovered that the incidence of infertility jumped 177 per cent between 1965 and 1982. Couples who find themselves unable to conceive are under enormous strain – feeling inadequate, their self-image and sexuality can go right down.

I can't make any promises, but I can tell you some success stories about nature's essential oils and their effect on fertility – and give some childless couples hope. Some couples, unfortunately, have a serious physiological problem – in women the most common problem is a blockage of the Fallopian tubes – and in these cases the essential oils can offer no remedy.

However, if you and your partner have been medically examined and been assured that there is no physiological reason behind your infertility, the essential oils may be able to help by working in two ways. First, we can overcome the 'catch-22' situation – the more desperate we are to conceive, the less this is likely to happen, because the avenues to conception get constricted, as it were, by our extreme tension. We need to relax and the essential oils are marvellous for this. Secondly, some essential oils have phytohormonal properties – plant hormones – which imitate our own.

Dr Jean Valnet, much revered in France as a leading light in phytotherapy – a branch of medicine very widespread in Europe – states that the essential oils that contain hormonal properties have a balancing effect on the endocrine glands, operating by dynamizing and giving the glands a new impetus, rather than taking over the functions of deficient glands. The application of essential oils, then, is seen as a form of physiological excitation therapy.

Female sterility is more likely to be due to the deficiency of a pituitary gland hormone than because the ovaries themselves are incapable of releasing ova for fertilization – we need to get the hormonal balance right. Oestrogens determine the female sexual cycle, on which fertility depends, and studies have shown that a woman increases her chances of becoming pregnant if that cycle is regular.

Research at the Monell Chemical Senses Center and the University of Pennsylvania in the USA has shown that male armpit secretions can influence the regularity of women's menstrual cycles, and so, strange as it may seem, one of the first things your partner can do is

151

throw away his deodorant! Meanwhile, research at Sonoma State Hospital in Eldridge, California has proved what generations of women have observed – women living or working together slowly synchronize their menstruation. This is known as the McClintock effect. Perhaps you should ask your sister to come and stay for a few months if her monthly cycle is regular. By the same token, if your cycle isn't regular, perhaps it's because you're working with a woman who has irregular periods, and you need to change offices!

You should aim to make love on the day that ovulation occurs – two weeks before the next period is due. If your partner's sperm count is low or the sperm aren't too mobile, he should avoid ejaculating for a few days before you have sex when ovulation is due.

Certain plants should be avoided because they produce an effect not conducive to conception. Yams, soya bean, sisal and fenugreek, for example, are all natural sources of 'sapogenin'. This is converted into sex hormones which are used in the birth-control pill. It is also used in the production of steroids such as cortisone. Clearly, if you want to conceive, it is sensible to avoid soya bean products and yams, and it should come as no surprise that although some of nature's products deter conception, some of them also promote it.

There are so many factors in successful conception – from the incidence of ovulation, through the mobility of the cilia within the Fallopian tube, to many other physiological processes – and it is by no means easy to understand why essential oil treatments can be successful. However, there seems to be some poetic justice in the fact that much of the essential oil of a plant is used to facilitate fertilization.

Mrs L. did not come to me because of childlessness, but because of the stress that was its result. She had been married for several years and both she and her husband were desperate for a child. Mrs L.'s stress manifested itself as profuse perspiration, and I included in her treatment, sage, which is the classic remedy used by professionals in the treatment of excessive perspiration, and also happens to be one of the essential oils that contains a great deal of the phytohormone that imitates oestrogen. Treatment lasted several months and over this period her perspiration problem disappeared and her confidence in herself returned. I waited to see if the treatment had had any positive 'side effects' and, sure enough, three months later she phoned, overjoyed, to tell me that she was pregnant. Years of trying for a baby were over. I have no way of being certain that it was my treatment that made Mrs L. able to conceive, but my case book gives me reason to think that nature's essential oils could have been responsible.

Mr J., for example, came to see me for arthritis but his major concern was to get his twenty-eight-year-old wife pregnant. Although I'm sure Mr J. would deny it, he looked to me about sixty-five to seventy years old and was worried that, after three years of trying, he wasn't able to follow in his grandfather's footsteps and sire many children well into his eighties. I explained to him that I was not a fertility specialist but he had tried everything, he told me, and was desperate. I treated his arthritis and also gave him relaxation and fertility treatment oils for both him and his wife to use at home. With instructions and oils in his pocket, he left. Eighteen months later I received a phone call, 'I've been feeling guilty about not calling you to let you know how we got on,' he said, 'but I have a son and we're all three very happy.'

Very many aromatherapy patients have had similar experiences and there are several physiological reasons to suppose that the essential oils could have been responsible – their relaxant properties, their imitation of human sexual hormones, their circulation and immune system stimulating properties, amongst others. In total, essential oils synchronize the body's natural rhythms and the subsequent natural balance allows the body to perform this most natural of functions. I repeat, I cannot make promises – all I can do is pass on my experience and information and wish you all success.

Oils for Women which Imitate the Hormone Oestrogen

Cypress	*Nutmeg*	*Oregano*
Clary-sage	*Anis vert*	*Basil*
Sage	*Angelica*	*Calendula*
Savory	*Cajeput*	*Star anise*
Parsley	*Coriander*	*Hop*
Thyme	*Geranium*	*Chamomile Roman*
Borneol	*Fennel*	

Other essential oils to try are those which are known empirically to aid the female reproductive system, as a uterine or ovarian tonic:

Uterine and Ovarian Tonics

Rose Bulgar ◇ *Melissa* ◇ *Geranium*

I would suggest that you follow a treatment of daily massage. Women can try any of the essential oils in all the lists above (men's come later), or try my special fertility synergistic blend.

Women's Fertility Synergistic Blend

Melissa	4 drops	*Make up a concentrate using these*
Rose Bulgar	7 drops	*proportions then use 1 drop per 1 ml*
Clary-sage	5 drops	*vegetable oil for massage*

You can make a massage oil using the synergistic blend above, a combination of the essential oils listed in this section of your own choice or, indeed, any one of those oils on their own. You could also benefit by including in your formula one of the essential oils with relaxant properties – see 'Sensuality and confidence' (page 121) to cross-check.

You can massage yourself or ask your partner to do it – over your abdomen, hips and lower back, just into the cleavage of the buttocks but not as far as the anus. A full-body massage can be a wonderfully relaxing prelude to lovemaking – relaxation is, in itself, a great help towards conception.

Three Women's Body Massage Oil Formulas to Aid Conception

Sage	10 drops	Rose Bulgar	8 drops	Anis vert	5 drops
Angelica	10 drops ◇	Geranium	16 drops ◇	Cypress	10 drops
Geranium	10 drops	Clary-sage	6 drops	Fennel	15 drops

Add any one formula to 30 ml of vegetable oil

Of course, it takes two to make a baby so here are some suggestions for men.

Essential Oils for Male Fertility

Cumin	Clary-sage	Sage
Angelica	Basil	

Two Men's Fertility Synergistic Blends

Cumin	10 drops		Angelica	9 drops
Clary-sage	8 drops	◇	Sage	8 drops
Basil	5 drops		Basil	6 drops

*Make a concentrate using these proportions, then use
1 drop per 1 ml of vegetable oil for massage or 2–4 drops in a bath*

A teaspoon of vegetable oil is quite sufficient for a massage and to this you add five drops of concentrate. Massage or rub the lower and upper abdominal muscles, pelvis and lower back area where the nerves to the gonads lie in the vertebrae (for the therapist: lumbar regions 4 and 3) – just into the crease of the buttocks, but not as far as the anus. Massaging these areas will stimulate the production of sperm.

The synergistic blend formulas will stimulate the whole body as well – after all, sperm may be produced in the gonads but the health of the whole body is important. Alternatively, make your own blend using the oils listed above, or on their own.

There is only empirical, but as yet no scientific, proof of the effectiveness of essential oil and aromatherapy methods of treating infertility; however, whether you try using essential oils before or after running the gamut of expensive hospital or clinic routines, what have you got to lose?

OILS TO GET IN SHAPE WITH

It's difficult to feel sensual and at ease in bed if you're so unhappy with your naked body that you're frightened to take off your clothes in front of your lover. We all know what the 'perfect' woman looks like – we see her and her friends every day on a hundred advertising billboards. Even so-called 'liberated' women's magazines illustrate their articles about 'realizing the real you' with photographs of women with figures that definitely don't look like the real you. It can be demoralizing getting up and out of bed, let alone getting undressed and into bed!

There are a number of ways that nature's essential oils can help you to shape up your body, but no oil can do it on its own – you need to exercise and diet as well. What the oils can do, however – and to great effect – is speed up the elimination process, detoxify the body and tone up the flab. I have patients who swear by my formulas and wouldn't be without them.

When Joan came to see me she was in a wretched state. She was a nurse on a geriatric ward, used to lifting heavy people all day, and her legs were strong and sturdy but her lower half was not its ideal shape. Joan had met a man she absolutely adored but was embarrassed to make love with him because of her figure. She was determined to lose weight from her thighs and backside. She'd already tried umpteen different diets and done all manner of exercise from aerobics to weight training, but although she'd lost the excess weight from her face, bust and arms, the weight would not shift from her thighs and buttocks. Her problem wasn't so much fat, but hard lumps of cellulite all over her buttocks and upper thighs. As we know, cellulite is not a pretty sight – horrible lumps of tissue underneath the skin, which forms pockets and pitted areas when the fat is pinched.

Cellulite starts to form in pockets of fat when an overworked system slows down the elimination process. Areas of the body become unable to remove water and toxic wastes so the tissue thickens, hardens and you're left with puffy, bulging areas of skin that look like orange peel. There are many reasons for cellulite, including fatigue, lack of exercise, constipation, bad circulation, indulgence in toxic foods and problems with the digestive tract.

Although cellulite is sometimes thought to be an inevitable part of being a woman because of our oestrogen level, it affects men, too, and apart from the hormonal factor, is largely the result of poisons in the body being trapped in the fluid that surrounds all body cells, the interstitial fluid. We need to attack it on all fronts, starting with diet.

The first thing to do is change to a wholefood diet, eat lots of fresh fruit and vegetables and drink plenty of spring water – at least two pints a day. Cut out all the toxic drinks like alcohol, coffee and tea (although herb teas are fine, especially fennel and nettle) and say no to dairy products like milk, cream, butter and cheese. Eat plenty of raw vegetables and salads and avoid red meat.

Start deep breathing exercises as these increase the level of oxygen in your blood which helps eliminate the trapped toxic debris. Regular deep breathing not only fights cellulite but helps your sex life too. Physical exercise, even if only gentle, is vital because it stimulates the system and aids the elimination of those terrible toxins. Make sure the bowels are clear and avoid constipation. All of this will make you feel healthier as well as getting rid of extra pounds.

The next front in the battle is self-massage. Using the following formulas, or any of the Cellulite Eliminator oils, add a total of thirty drops to 30 ml of a fine vegetable oil. I recommend hazelnut or grapeseed for their penetrative properties, although any light vegetable or nut oil will do. Rub firmly into the fatty areas, trying to promote circulation.

The Cellulite Eliminator Oils

Oregano	Juniper
Thyme	Fennel
Lemon	Cypress
Grapefruit	Celery

Self-massage of the cellulite areas using nature's essential oils is an excellent method, but use the massage oil as you would any body-oil – after a bath or shower, or better still, after a session at the gym. Whichever way you use them, make sure it's at least twice a day for three weeks. In addition, you should have a daily essential oil bath, using a total of six drops.

Three Cellulite Eliminator Body Massage Formulas

Oregano	6 drops	Thyme	8 drops	Fennel	8 drops
Lemon	10 drops ◇	Celery	10 drops ◇	Cypress	10 drops
Juniper	14 drops	Grapefruit	12 drops	Lemon	12 drops

Joan followed my instructions to the letter – cutting out coffee and tea, sticking to the detoxifying diet, exercising and applying the essential oil formulas I gave her to use at home. The terrible toxins in her cellulite got flushed out and slowly but surely her lumps and bumps went. She was delighted to find that underneath the unsightly cellulite her legs and buttocks began to take on a nice sleek look. She could never have been a model, but Joan was finally in very good shape nonetheless, and with her new-found confidence the sensuous Aromantic woman in her blossomed. Now, she was ready for love.

If your bone structure is on the large side, you can still look good. Nature doesn't make us all the same shape and size, and it would be very boring if we were. However, nature did intend us to be healthy and take care of the body she gave us. If you have no cellulite but want to improve your body shape, the same thing applies - you must exercise – and the essential oils of nature can help you to tone up, too. Although using these oils won't miraculously turn you into a cover-girl (unless you're halfway there already, lucky you!) I think you'll be pretty pleased with the results.

Keep-in-Shape Oils

Lemongrass	Cedarwood
Lavender	Lime
Rosemary	Pettigraine

Three Keep-in-Shape Body Massage Formulas

Lemongrass	15 drops	◇	Rosemary	15 drops	◇	Cedarwood	15 drops
Pettigraine	15 drops		Lavender	15 drops		Lime	15 drops

Diluted in a base-oil

Massage the oil firmly into the areas that you want to tone up at least once a day, including after you bathe or shower. Keep this routine up for at least a week and you will see results. The inner thighs respond particularly well to rosemary and lavender. Using the same combinations of two essential oils as you would for the massage oil, you can also add three drops of each (x 2) to baths.

159

The female body is subject to the dictates of fashion perhaps most especially in the area of the breasts. Lucky for us if we happen to be the right size at the right time!

Before you go thinking that this obsession with having 'perfect' breasts is something new, a product of the commercial age, you might be interested to know that four thousand years ago, in ancient Egypt, women baked the seeds of a pretty, delicate blue flower, love-in-a-mist (*Nigella damascena*), in bread as they thought it would increase their breast size. They also used to hang the seeds in a little cloth bag between their breasts, where the warmth of their bodies would release the fragrance.

Apparently, women have never been satisfied with their breast size! Indeed, to many, breasts have been the sign, *par excellence*, of femininity. While it's impossible to change the shape and size of your bust simply by using essential oils, they can certainly aid any exercise pattern you may be using.

I first developed my breast-toning formulas in response to a request from June, who not only had no breasts to speak of but an inverted nipple as well. She felt very conscious of the fact that she didn't look like the girls in centre spreads, and although it hadn't affected her relationships with men, she felt threatened and uncomfortable in the company of other women.

June had decided to buy herself a bust exerciser that built up the pectoral muscles which, in turn, gives the impression that the breasts are larger. I made up a formula for her to use at the same time which included several essential oils that stimulate the female hormone, oestrogen. To both our amazements, the fatty tissue of the breast increased as well! Since then I've used the formula with great success many times. It stimulates the breast tissue, firming and – with exercise – increases the size of the breast. Don't think you'll become another Dolly Parton, but your natural form can be increased and rounded.

The essential oils and formulas listed below,

however, should not be used by women who are pregnant or breastfeeding. These women aren't alone – they are two people and that little person, the baby, must be treated like a separate person with quite different needs. Remember, any oil you use, baby will get too. Women who are breastfeeding are often the most concerned to tone up and reshape their breasts at this time, but they should never use any essential oils whatsoever on the breasts while nursing baby. They just have to be patient and use the formulas here when the breastfeeding period is over. To them, I say that I'm sorry if this advice is disappointing, but your breasts' first function is to feed your baby, not look good in the mirror, and your man, I'm sure, loves the shape of your breasts and delights in their function. Enjoy your breastfeeding now and enjoy using the breast-toning oils later!

Here are the essential oils and formulas for firming and enlarging the breasts.

Breast-enlarging Oils

Fennel	Angelica	Lemongrass
Clary-sage	Geranium	Hop
Sage	Cypress	Parsley

Three Breast-enlarging Formulas

Fenugreek	14 drops	Fennel	10 drops	Angelica	10 drops
Clary-sage	10 drops ◇	Clary-sage	10 drops ◇	Clary-sage	10 drops
Geranium	6 drops	Geranium	10 drops	Hop	10 drops

Use any of these formulas, make up your own, or use a single oil from the list above to a total of thirty drops per 30 ml of vegetable oil. Massage the flesh of the breasts, not the nipple or areola, in a movement I call the Charleston Rub, because it looks like the hand movements of the dance – put a little oil on both hands and using them both at the same time, rub in circular movements outwards towards the underarms. Your left hand should be moving clockwise around the breast and your right hand, anticlockwise. Do this daily.

Lemongrass used on its own will lift and tone the tissue if persevered with. Geranium is reported to be very rich in phytohormones, plant hormones which are similar to the human hormones responsible for, amongst other things, the development of the breasts. Fenugreek, although not such a good source of phyto-hormones, has been used throughout history to encourage lactation and roundness of the breasts – but as I have already said, don't use any of these oils and formulas if you're breastfeeding (or pregnant). Also, fenugreek should not be used if you're trying to conceive (see 'Fertility').

In his book *The Practice of Aromatherapy*, Dr Jean Valnet recommends the use of anise, fennel, carraway and lemongrass to increase the size of breasts and I would suggest that you use them in equal proportions, seven drops of each of the four oils in 30 ml of vegetable oil.

Although the essential oils do work wonders in aiding the toning and shaping of the body, remember, this cannot be accomplished without some self-help from you in the form of exercise and diet. What we put inside will very much determine what we look like on the outside. Onion, for example, is well known for normalizing glandular imbalance and helping dieters – so long as the dieter uses them in clear onion soup rather than fried onion rings!

5

Aromantic Man

HOW TO BECOME THE AROMANTIC MAN

A man's life is full of pressure. Society urges him to 'get on' and 'achieve' – euphemisms for making money. Glossy billboard advertising makes it quite clear that if a 'real' man eats quiche, he also eats caviar and drives a Porsche! This is a world in which men gain respect by being 'winners' rather than 'losers'.

As if all this weren't enough, when a man gets into bed there's more pressure – the pressure to perform. It doesn't matter that his woman doesn't overtly lay pressure on him: that is hardly necessary in a world which sees the act of lovemaking as something a man either does well or badly and which women 'respond' to. A man could have the most sensitive and equal-minded woman in the world, but that can't obliterate years of subtle programming from a miscellany of sources.

All too often, then, it isn't a real 'man' who gets into bed, but an overloaded robot, chock–full of images and expectations that have nothing to do with him himself, but with everyone else – from his parents, peers and partner to the publicists of machismo. He may even wish that his penis would behave like an extension of the mechanical robot he has become – but it doesn't. The sensitivity of the penis, exasperating as it may sometimes be, is in fact man's saving grace – it reminds us all that man is a sensitive human being.

The Aromantic man is neither a super-robot nor oversensitive and pressurized. Aromantic man is the man who has found himself and refound his natural, God-given self-confidence and strength. Men were designed to make love! There is no need to worry about your capacity and performance, only the need to realize your true potential, and enjoy.

You don't have to worry that there's something rather indulgent about becoming an Aromantic man – nature's essential oils come highly recommended. In the Bible, Proverbs 27:9, we're told, 'Ointment and perfume rejoice the heart: so doth the sweetness of a man's friend by hearty counsel' and in Revelation 5:8, we're told that 'vials full of odours' are 'the prayers of saints'.

The spiritual link is probably most widely known in the giving of frankincense and myrrh to baby Jesus by two of the three wise men at Bethlehem. Frankincense is a profoundly spiritual oil and myrrh is a healing agent, due to its anti-bacterial properties. Aromantics still use these and other essential oils today. According to Eugene Rimmel, the prophet Mahomet professed a great fondness for essential oils and resins, saying that what his heart enjoyed most in this world were children, women and perfumes. Certainly, in the Islamic paradise, the *Djennet Firdous*, perfumes formed a conspicuous part. Islamic tradition has it that the white rose was created from Mahomet's sweat as he rose to heaven; the red rose grew where Gabriel's sweat dropped to the ground; and the yellow rose sprung up where the sweat of El-Burák (the animal that carried Mahomet from Mecca to Jerusalem) fell on the ground. Whatever the truth behind historical anecdote, there is hardly a religious group operating today that does not include aromatics in their rituals.

The Egyptian civilization spanned from around 4236 BC, the first year of their calendar, to 30 BC when Cleopatra and Antony committed suicide and Octavian declared Egypt a Roman province and, as you'd expect, over this four-thousand-year period the use of nature's essential oils went through some changes. At first, only pharaohs were considered close enough to the divine to use the oils, which were guarded by the priests. The pharaohs would give their precious oils as gifts to men who had performed some outstanding social deed, rather as our leaders award medals today. By 2450 BC Phah-Hotep was telling Egyptian men the proper way to conduct their marriages: 'If thou art a man of standing thou shouldst fill her belly, clothe her back and ointment is the prescription of her body.' (Being Aromantic isn't new!) By around AD 1175 when Rameses III was trying to get the necropolis built at Thebes, the workers were going on strike because they weren't getting the food and 'ointments' they had been promised.

You don't have to worry that nature's essential oils are 'cissy'. The Roman soldiers (who definitely didn't eat quiche!) were also fond of their 'ointments'. Indeed, according to Juvenal no fashionable Roman officer would go to war without them. (Julius Caesar preferred his soldiers to smell of garlic – and we all know what happened to him!) In the latter Roman period the flags and standards of the army were sprinkled with perfume. When the victorious soldiers arrived home they were showered with flowers and would then, no doubt, retire to the steam baths for a freshen-up before the orgy. Naturally, they would insist on their favourite fragrances being added to the bath water and included in their massage oils. Indeed, it's even reported that the Romans rubbed their horses and dogs with scented ointment. If this sounds far-fetched, consider the fact that the Indians used to give female elephants a perfumed rubdown after their baths – to inflame the bull elephants to passion!

Alexander the Great was certainly not short of

machismo, and yet when he and his army marched across the landscape towards India in 329 BC, the geographer, Strabo, recorded the fact that they gathered branches of myrrh-producing trees and various aromatic grasses to make the thatched roofs of their tents – to make them sleep comfortably in a sweet atmosphere. According to Athenaeus, Alexander's floor was sprinkled with exquisite perfumes and he used fragrant resins and myrrh, along with other kinds of incense. So extravagant was Alexander's use of incense that he incurred criticism from his old tutor, Leonidas, who told him 'so to worship when he had conquered the countries that produced the frankincense'. Perhaps it was this comment that drove Alexander to conquer Arabia, for when he had done so he shipped a cargo of frankincense and myrrh back to Leonidas! But Alexander had not always been so aroma-minded. When he had vanquished Darius at the battle of Arbela, one of the things he found in Darius's tent was 'precious aromatics' – which Alexander threw out with contempt. Only later, after travelling in Asia, did he come to realize and appreciate their value.

To the Indians, as to the Hebrews and ancient Egyptians, nature's essential oils were considered to be the special fragrances of the gods. Of course, the Indian kings and emperors – like rulers everywhere and at all times – liked to luxuriate in the aromatic 'ointments'. In AD 1130 the Sanskrit author Someshvara, described the ideal bath for the ruler. After being washed by beautiful attendants, his hair and scalp should be washed with the fragrant pulp of *amalaka*, and then rinsed. Then athletes should massage the whole body before a final fragrant oil was put on by female attendants. This last preparation consisted of a sesame oil base, perfumed with jasmine, coriander, cardamom, basil, costus, pandanus, agarwood, pine saffron, champac and clove. Only now was the king ready to face the day. Fourteen hundred years earlier, a marvellous picture of an Indian emperor's lifestyle was painted by the Greek ambassador, Megasthenes, who visited Chandragupta: the emperor sits listening to the complaints of his subjects while his feet are massaged with scented oils, his hair was combed and his body massaged with wooden rollers.

Such a scene wouldn't have come as much of a shock to Megasthenes because, back home in Athens, he would have been used to going to high-class social gatherings where the guests were massaged by slaves using aromatic oils. Being such a poetic folk, the ancient Greeks added perfume to their fountains when guests were due, and perhaps as Aromantics use water bowls today – to help their guests relax. Not that everyone agreed with all this indulgence. Socrates disapproved of perfumes because 'there is the same smell in a slave and a gentleman'!

Economists might like to note that when China suffered a balance of payments crisis in AD 970 the government invented a silk and paper currency which they impregnated with perfume to give the money a wider appeal! You see, nothing much is new – we just find different ways to deal with the same problems.

There was a time in the twentieth century when men's need of aroma was dismissed scornfully, but not now. NASA quickly realized that spacemen soon develop a desperate need for aroma in their super-technical, metallic spaceships. The American astronauts would pass lemon-scented 'handiwipes' to each other to share the whiff before using them to wipe the inside of their helmets to let the aroma hang around them during the long space flight. The old Soviet Union used to have a very sophisticated programme of research into the emotional effects of nature's essential oils and for many years sent their astronauts into the wide blue yonder with little phials of aroma – scents to allay emotional deprivation. The modern world has finally awoken to the emotional effects of aroma.

Nature's essential oils aren't just about the sweet smell of perfume nor, indeed, just about their medicinal effects, which are impressive (a fact the Roman soldiers no doubt considered). What we're talking about here are substances which reach beyond the physical and into the limbic system, the emotional control box, and beyond even that – into your soul.

Frankincense is traditionally the substance used in churches – and this is why: it brings enlightenment and protects you from the materialistic world while releasing your subconscious and uplifting your spirit. Sandalwood, on the other hand, helps you to make peace with the world. It's a profoundly masculine oil, sedative, seductive, sweet, rich and warm. Vetiver is sexually arousing and strengthening, earthy and positive in a no-nonsense way. Vetiver releases deeply felt tensions and fears – it's for getting what you want out of life. Basil is a go-getter too, but in a different way – it stimulates, sharpens the senses, clarifies the intellect, helps you to concentrate and strengthens the nerves.

When you become the Aromantic man, you'll understand why men throughout history have held nature's essential oils in such high esteem. You too will share the benefits enjoyed by kings, emperors and the heroes of history, but you'll have the added advantage of a far wider variety of precious oils, thanks to our sophisticated communication and transportation systems.

In this chapter I shall be giving you my exclusive formulas to help you to become the Aromantic man. You will be vibrating with the joys of spring, in control of your erection and ejaculation, no longer worn down by anxiety, stress and tension, or worn out by muscular fatigue; we'll be looking at formulas to help the older man too.

The Especially Masculine Oils

Ambrette ◆ Anis vert ◆ Basil ◆ Bay ◆ Benzoin
Bergamot ◆ Black pepper ◆ Bois de rose ◆ Cardamom
Cedarwood ◆ Cinnamon ◆ Clary-sage ◆ Cumin
Frankincense ◆ Geranium ◆ Ginger ◆ Jasmine ◆ Lemon
Mace ◆ Melissa ◆ Mimosa ◆ Myrrh ◆ Narcissus
Orange ◆ Palma rosa ◆ Patchouli ◆ Pine ◆ Sandalwood
Vanilla ◆ Vetiver

GERANIUM is for adjusting the mood and regenerating the positive effects of life while dispelling anxieties and shutting the door on apprehension. It elevates the intimate.

MACE is soft, warm and sultry. It's gently evocative but can be delusive. Definitely for arousing more than the imagination!

PATCHOULI is like the warm earth. It accentuates the masculine and reaches deep into the emotions. Stimulating and persistent, yet voluptuous and suggestive like ancient eroticism.

ANIS VERT is alive and distinct. It stimulates the physical while emphasizing positivity.

BASIL is stimulating and go-getting. It sharpens the senses and concentration, clarifying the intellect while strengthening the nerves.

CARDAMOM is spicy. It lightly stimulates the mind into clarity. Yet it is profoundly sexual in nature, evoking the erotic nature of man. For the sensuous, clear thinker.

AMBRETTE is animalistic. Like a warm responsive body it stimulates the sexual man, yet gently and sweetly takes the edge off events.

SANDALWOOD is a profoundly masculine oil, seda-tive and seductive. It helps you make peace with the world and your woman. It's sweet, rich and warm.

BAY has been for centuries presented to heroes and the victors of battle. It is distinctive and sexually arrogant. It stimulates imaginative decisions. Not for the submissive!

BLACK PEPPER has stamina and strength like the heroes of legend. It's peppery, hot and dry and can stimulate your mind and body into action. It seeks out hidden anger and frustration and precociously defrosts the frozen-hearted.

JASMINE is the mistress of the night, bringing out man's desire and fantasies while accentuating the feminine and stimulating the seduction!

BOIS DE ROSE is for when you feel neglected and abandoned. It's sweet and unemotional, brings tran-quillity and yet exhilarates the conscious mind.

NARCISSUS is earthy and hypnotic. It's deeply settling and relaxes a depressive state, bringing a vitalizing calm, desirous and sensual.

MIMOSA is like the new spring growth. It's powerful and penetrating, renewing the sense of well-being, and deeply alluring. It helps to open the lines of communication in a relationship.

ORANGE is bright and lively, with a warm glow of copper. It disperses the fear of the unknown and helps release obsessions, creating a positive outlook, particularly with regard to emotional tangles.

VETIVER relaxes deeply felt tensions and fears. It's sexually arousing and strengthening, earthy and positive with a no-nonsense attitude. It's for getting what you want out of life.

MYRRH is smoky and musky, amplifying strength and courage; mysterious and seductive, filled with the passions of antiquity.

CUMIN is erotic, bizarre and evocative. It can powerfully stimulate the flow of bodily juices while warmly penetrating the senses of man and woman.

CEDARWOOD gives you a harmonious strength and fortitude. It releases tension and aggression and relaxes the analytical mind.

MELISSA is vivacious and provocative, like a woman in love. It embraces the perilous with a calm sensitivity, revitalizing the inner man.

FRANKINCENSE protects you from the materialistic world. It brings enlightenment, releasing subconscious stress and uplifting the spirit.

BERGAMOT is sharply keen to the senses and helps you get directly in control with composure and distinction.

VANILLA is familiar and consoling, offers safety from the harsh blows of life. It unleashes deeply felt emotions and hidden sensuality.

PINE is the philosopher. It brings peace and wisdom yet activates your energy. For the apathetic and depressed. It can invigorate the mind like a walk through a snow-covered pine forest.

GINGER is arousing and warm, fortifying and opulent, inviting and satisfying.

CLARY-SAGE is masculine and seductive, warm and desirous. Like an opiate, yet forceful.

PALMA ROSA is light and sweet. It lightly lifts the senses and clarifies the thoughts.

CINNAMON is stimulating and refreshing, sensually calming the nerves and tension while diminishing the harshness of the day. To steady the nerves and stimulate the senses.

BENZOIN wraps you up, like having a shield against the events of the day. It releases long forgotten tensions and resentments enabling you to relax into higher awareness.

LEMON is for the humourless and indecisive. It relaxes yet stimulates. It's clean, fresh and lively but still sedating; it's equally good for waking up and getting to sleep.

But before we take a closer look at nature's essential oils and how they can help you, let's first ask ourselves what it means to be a sexual man today. There's no doubt that the male and female experience of sex is different – not necessarily emotionally, but in terms of expectations and pressures. For example, imagine what would happen if a man in a happy, steady sexual relationship suddenly went off sex for no apparent reason and this disinterest lasted for several months. The chances are that before long, he, his partner, the doctor and the psychiatrist would begin to suspect that he was becoming impotent. Yet when precisely this happened to a girlfriend of mine, Gloria, she could say 'I've just gone off sex' without any fear or worry, just slight bemusement. Nobody is concerned that Gloria has changed from a highly sexed woman into a 'frigid' one, and really, why should they be? Sex doesn't come in daily, weekly or monthly rationed portions. We can go through whole periods of time highly charged sexually or with hardly any sexual feeling at all, and the distinction doesn't necessarily relate to partner availability or our degree of love for them. A man, too, should be able to take 'time off' occasionally, but because we are all so worried about the spectre of impotency, he just has to keep going whether he really feels like it or not. This form of performance pressure makes sex a duty – a job, not a joy – and may partly account for the fact that sometimes men ejaculate, but feel very little. Men fake orgasms too! Perhaps, before we go any further, we should ask, 'What is male orgasm?' Although in most men's experience orgasm and ejaculation occur at one and the same time, they are in fact two separate physical processes. Sex therapist Bernie Zilbergeld defines orgasm as having very pleasurable feelings, and ejaculation as the physical process involved when the semen is propelled through the penis and makes the point that these two processes can occur without each other. Not only can a man ejaculate but feel no pleasure, he can feel the pleasure of orgasm without ejaculating. This last option is obviously the better and is indeed the goal of Chinese and Indian sexual training of men, the former for medicinal reasons and the latter for spiritual ones. Zilbergeld records that some modern-day men have also trained themselves and report being able to have multiple orgasms like women. Others have very high peaks of feeling which, Zilbergeld speculates, would be called orgasms if the men could shake off the 'indoctrination' that orgasm only occurs with pelvic contraction and ejaculation.

It's taken women years to come to the understanding that their orgasmic response may be mild, multiple, clitoral, vaginal, vulval, blended, G-spot, ejaculatory or uterine (to mention just some of the classifications currently under discussion) and that no type is 'better' than another. Surely, as male orgasm does not equate physically with ejaculation, men can begin to think of their orgasmic response patterns in the same way – as colours of the rainbow, with the diversity of colour, rather than just a single colour, being the real beauty. In other words, let's explore!

Sex is a very complex subject and it isn't possible to understand it simply in terms of mechanics or muscular contractions at 0.8 second intervals! Sex is about chemistry, desire, electricity, and all sorts of things that have nothing to do with bare flesh, and yet men are goal-driven into getting a woman's flesh bare as soon as possible, penetrating her and ejaculating. The strange thing about this idea is, that in the rush all the magical, energy-packed moments that preceded the apparent 'goal' get trampled underfoot, like so much garbage at a crowded football match. Poor old magic, you've got to feel sorry for it!

You only need one or two drops of essential oil, tiny an amount as that may sound, and they're best used in candles. The word 'perfume' derives from the Latin 'per fumin' – by smoke – and this ancient technique takes full advantage of the fact that the essential oils release their tiny but powerful molecules more quickly and with increased force when exposed to heat. Put a drop inside the candle, not on the wick, but on the melted wax before it dribbles down. You can put the oil in place before the expected 'magic moments' and light up when the time seems right, releasing a delightful, soft aroma into the air. You can also use a room diffuser.

Here then is the first group of oils and formulas. Use them when you want to amplify the sexual tension that happens before sex – when the electricity between you is like a charge in the atmosphere, when a look is no longer a look but an exciting, meaningful exchange between two souls and when an accidental touch sends shivers through you both. This is a special time, worth luxuriating in and enjoying to the full.

Magic Moment Oils

Clary-sage	◀ *Used alone*	Geranium
Jasmine	*or mix*	Lemon
	with ▶	Rose Maroc
		Hyacinth

Four Magic Moment Synergistic Blends

Clary-sage	3 drops		Clary-sage	3 drops
Geranium	1 drop	◇	Lemon	1 drop

Clary-sage	10 drops		Jasmine	3 drops
Geranium	4 drops	◇	Verbena	2 drops
Lemon	2 drops			

To this last synergistic blend on the left, you can add two drops of frankincense for a special, spiritual edge.

It is best not to use the magic moment candles over dinner as taste and smell are so inextricably linked that it's hard to tell one from the other. Why spoil either? Have coffee, inhale the aroma of your good brandy, then light the magic moment candle to experience a 'total olfactory banquet'! A good oil to use now is cardamom which is an excellent digestive aid, or make a synergistic blend using three drops of cardamom and one of jonquil.

Whether you make an overt sexual advance towards your ladyfriend during these magic moments is entirely up to you, but don't be bullied into it by the performance pressure of male 'pride'. The 'hunter and prey' syndrome gets tiring for men and women alike and she'll probably enjoy the respite. She won't go home feeling flat, but high, and will remember this unusual occasion as sexy and sensual and altogether delightful. Of course, she could make an advance herself, and if she wants you but doesn't make a move, she may need to develop her sexual initiative skills; so if you think about it that way, you're really doing her a favour by tantalizing her. She'll get home and kick herself; 'I should have made a pass, I really should'. In any case, by the next time you see each other her desire level will be right up – and Aromantic man will be ready for her!

THE AROMANTIC MAN, *APRÈS L'AMOUR*

I'm sorry to say that some men come in for criticism for their actions after lovemaking. Actually, when I say actions, I mean non-actions! Women tell me time and time again, 'He's so romantic when he wants sex, then as soon as he comes he turns his back and goes to sleep'.

Partly, the problem stems from the fact that many women don't understand that men have a 'refractory period' after ejaculatory orgasm, and that this period increases with age. Clinically speaking, this is the length of time during which a man cannot again ejaculate, although in practice it tends to be the time during which he has no further interest in sex. During puberty the refractory period lasts a mere couple of seconds to one minute, but by late middle age it could

176

be twelve hours. A woman can easily interpret her man's increasing lack of interest in her after his orgasm as a lack of love when, in fact, it's just that his refractory period is increasing with the years.

The ejaculatory orgasm is profoundly tiring and this too is an experience many women don't understand. They're ready for cuddling, talking and touching – reaffirming love for each other – and he's asleep! She may think, 'Well, I've had a hard day too and I haven't fallen asleep. Maybe he doesn't want to cuddle and be close; perhaps he doesn't love me any more.' This could be the time when seeds are sown for those arguments that appear out of nowhere.

Perhaps, too, much of the problem stems from the idea that all lovemaking should end in intercourse. If a man knows that he won't want sex again, and thinks cuddles should lead inexorably to intercourse, he'll obviously turn his back so that she gets the message. Sometimes it may seem easier for him to upset his wife than admit that his needs have changed. But it isn't just older men who fail to appreciate what a special time *après l'amour* can be.

The sensation of touch can be tremendously heightened *après l'amour*, when all the nerves of the body have just had a 'tonic' and the chemicals of ecstasy are still floating around. Cuddling now is no ordinary cuddling – it's two people completely relaxed and secure in their love for each other luxuriating in the feeling of being as one. Subjects that could not be broached before sex are easier raised when we've just proved our acceptance of the partner and confirmed our affection and love. *Après l'amour* is no time for war!

If you're too exhausted at the end of the day for anything more than lovemaking and sleep, carve out some other time in your busy schedule for sharing intimacy. Go to bed earlier or make love on a Saturday or Sunday and have an *après l'amour* lie-in. Your sexual relationship is probably the most important relationship you have, and 'sexual' isn't just about intercourse but about tenderness, togetherness, touch, communication and enjoying the security of each other's warmth. So find time to share these things and let your woman know that she is special.

In the Aromantic woman's *Après l'amour* section (page 118) you'll find the essential oils for accentuating the romantic and erotic, opening up the channels of communication, balancing out the emotions, and the stimulating oils for men (if she starts to give you a back-rub after you next make love, you'll know what's going on). And you could rub her back, too – most women love this. It may induce sleep in her and an erection in you and, if so, intercourse now could be special for her because the dreamy state as she enters sleep can produce a highly erotic orgasm (and it's worth noting that ancient Indian love manuals suggested that women with low sexual response should make love more often on the same day). But you don't have to have intercourse if you find that you have an erection now – just enjoy the sensations of 'purposeless tension', as the Indian sages would say. Simply enjoy being alive and well!

You can use one of the oils and methods described in the woman's section or give your special lady a gentle back-rub using the oils below, paying particular attention to the lower half of her back.

Après l'amour Oils

Group 1		Group 2
Ylang-ylang	Take one from each group	Nutmeg
Jasmine	Mix together in equal	Tonka bean
Palma rosa	proportions, to 30 drops, then	Opopanax
Orange	add to 30 ml of vegetable oil	Frankincense

Below are some examples, using the proportions you need for one back-rub application.

Three *Après l'amour* Ladies' Rubs

Ylang-ylang 1 drop ◄ *Add to 1 dessertspoon* ► *Palma rosa 1 drop*
Tonka bean 1 drop   *of vegetable oil*   *Nutmeg 1 drop*
▼

| *Jasmine* | *1 drop* |
| *Frankincense* | *1 drop* |

HOW TO RELEASE YOUR SEXUAL VIBRATION

The *real* you was designed to make love. And I do mean *make* love. The expression 'relief of tension' which is so prevalent in our society today is symptomatic of the fact that we're under so much pressure we see sex as a necessary release of negativity instead of a positive generator of energy, like a battery we can plug into. Sex should be invigorating, not exhausting. We shouldn't think of it as a desperate 'relief' that stops us going crazy and saves our lives, but as something incredibly beautiful that makes life the understandable drama we can approach with a philosophical outlook, equanimity and humour.

Part of the problem is that we're spoiled for choice – which career path to take; which TV station to watch; where to live; who to talk to. In all the looking about we can forget to look inside – at us. Who are we? Who are you?

This section is about discovering the real you because your sexual vibration doesn't exist outside, it's inside, and we want to bring it out from within – with a little help from the essential oils.

So, let's forget about what we don't have and concentrate on what we do have. First, we have touch. Already today you've probably touched a hundred different textures – can you remember any of them? Right now, close your eyes and feel around. Really concentrate on the different textures you can feel: run your fingers over everything and register with super-awareness. Isn't it remarkable just how different everything feels from everything else?

Try every day, just for one minute, to increase your sensitivity to touch. If you were blind, you'd appreciate it a lot more. Try not to go through another day without registering touch, and tonight I want you to touch yourself as you've never touched yourself before – with appreciation. Close your eyes again and feel your face and hair. Even feel your eyelashes – aren't they sweet? Feel your skin all over – there are places where it's softer, hairier, where the muscles are firm and strong, where the flesh is fatty.

It's this same sensitive, appreciative form of touch that you'll later be applying to your partner. She is as unique as you. Nobody in this whole world feels like her. Close your eyes and run your fingertips over her body, aware of every nook and cranny you come across. Then, with the flat of your hand, feel the form, the shape of her. What does her stomach feel like? Or her back? She feels good, doesn't she?

Now open your eyes and look. Get close, as close as an insect, and you'll be surprised by what you see on this undulating landscape of wonder. Some men have been married to a woman for forty years and they couldn't even tell you where she has scars or moles. And some men never even look at their woman's vagina, and yet they put part of their own body into it day after day. What are they frightened of? This is a miracle you're looking at. This is the gateway to life. Now look at the gateway to her soul – her eyes. Don't just glance. Explore deep inside her eyes, searching out her character and personality. Go beyond 'look' – *see*!

Until we lose one of our senses, we just take them for granted. Some perfumers are so sensitive to smell, so trained and aware, they can tell a blonde from a brunette and a brunette from a redhead – with their eyes closed. Could you? Of course not, not now, but you could if you developed your sense of smell. So smell your woman's hair, her neck, chest and arms and try to lock her aromas into your memory. Then tomorrow, when you're at work, see if you can recall them.

Being sensuous helps to make a man or woman a good lover – aware, receptive and appreciative. The most famous lover of history, Don Juan, appreciated every one of his conquests and they loved him for it. Try to get in tune with your lover, on a closer vibration, and things will really hum.

Here then are some oils and formulas to help you become a sensuous man. They stimulate areas of the brain that relate to the senses and include some that contain molecules similar to human sexual hormonal secretions which will help you develop your sense of smell. And remember, smell isn't just about aesthetics; aroma goes directly to the brain and unlocks doors to emotion.

Use the oils in the bath or shower, on a source of heat in the room, or added to vegetable oil for a body-rub. Avoiding the genitals completely, rub the oil lightly over your lower abdomen and over your lower back – just into the cleavage of your buttocks but not as far as the anus.

The Sensuous Oils

Cumin
Ambrette
Geranium
Patchouli
Sandalwood

5 drops per teaspoon of vegetable oil

Or try one of my exclusive synergistic blend formulas.

Two Sensuous Man's Synergistic Blends

Ambrette	2 drops		Sandalwood	5 drops
Lemon	5 drops	◇	Geranium	3 drops
Black pepper	4 drops		Cumin	3 drops

Make a concentrate using these proportions,
then add 5 drops to 1 teaspoon of vegetable oil

Important though the sense of touch is, sexual vibration and, more specifically, a man's erection, does not depend upon it. Men who have spinal cord injuries where the brain can no longer perceive touch of the penis can still get an erection simply from thinking, seeing, hearing or smell. According to sex therapist, Avodah Offit, the research into this subject shows that sympathetic pathways are still operating and that with particular thoughts, sights, sounds or smells, these men can still function sexually despite their numbness in the genital region.

However, this isn't to say that physical problems don't cause trouble – they do. A man's sexual vibration may be stifled by stress-related illnesses, such as ulcers, depression, cancer and cardiac arrests; or by prostate gland problems, heart disease, high blood pressure, bronchial trouble, obesity, and alcohol and drugs, both illegal and legal. A low sexual vibration can be a symptom of a more serious physical condition and you may need a thorough medical check-up, or a frank discussion with your doctor about your libido and the possible side effects on it that any prescribed drugs may be having.

Low sexual vibration may merely be a side effect of a sluggish body, and men who have gone from a no-exercise lifestyle to a physical exercise programme certainly report an upturn in their sexual vibrancy when they do so. Arguments in a relationship don't help anything at all, including sex, and it could be that you both need some kind of counselling to jolt yourselves out of the blame-strain vortex. Notorious culprits in the suppression of sexual vibrancy are stress, tension, depression and overwork, some of which we deal with later. Boredom is often the underlying cause of relationship difficulties, but by the time you and the Aromantic woman have worked your way through this book, I can assure you that won't be a problem!

Clearly, there are many factors which could contribute to low sexual vibrancy, either alone or in conjunction with each other. You must take a good look at your life and decide where the problems are. Draw up a list of the possible culprits and tick off the ones that look relevant to your life. The essential oils of nature cannot be expected to provide solutions to all the culprits – lack of exercise or excess alcohol and food, for example. These are things you must decide to tackle yourself. But nature's essential oils can provide great help in other areas, so choose your oils from the lists below.

For Aromantic Man

Stimulants	Adaptogens: Stimulants/sedatives	Sedatives
Rosemary	Geranium	Sandalwood
Orange	Rose Maroc	Cedarwood
Melissa	Bois de rose	Cypress
Jasmine	Nutmeg	Bergamot

Sexual Stimulants

Ylang-ylang   *Please note that ylang-ylang*
Cumin   *in large doses can have*
Cistus   *the opposite effect*

Some essential oils are 'dual-purpose' in that they can treat two different types of problem, depending on the needs of the person. For example, lavender will perk you up in the morning if you feel sluggish but need the

183

stimulation and yet, at night, will sedate you if you're feeling tired but your mind is buzzing. The subtlety and paradoxical nature of essential oils can be difficult to understand until we remember that nature is herself paradoxical. You are nature too, don't forget, and the very fact of being sluggish but just awake, or buzzing and yet tired, are conditions that are paradoxical in themselves. The dual-purpose, 'adaptogen' essential oils will seek out and discover your real needs at any particular time, and will serve those needs. If you can't decide whether you need a stimulant or a sedative, choose an oil from the adaptogen list on page 183 and let your body tell you what it really wants.

The only thing you need now is time. Yes, I know you don't have any, but you don't need much and it's time well spent. Really, when you think about it, isn't part of the problem to do with the fact that, rather than your libido deserting you, you have deserted your libido? You need to pay libido some attention, too.

Plan a sexy evening with your partner – you don't have to spend a great deal of cash, just plan to go out and spend a little time together. Start your romantic day by running a bath, or having a shower if you prefer, and adding the essential oil to the bath water or to the sponge or face-cloth you use when you wash. Relax and inhale the vapour, close your eyes and think about your partner at their most sexual. Imagine how wonderful it could be later on. We're all very rushed in the morning, but start your day just five minutes earlier to allow yourself a relaxed soak, inhaling the vapour and allowing your mind to wander in this way. Throughout the day prepare your mind and nervous system for a sexual experience. How you do this depends on you and your imagination – take a favourite photo of your partner to work to remind yourself of what is to come or phone them at lunchtime and say, 'I love you'. No matter what's going on when you get home, sublimely ignore all negativity, take your partner out for a while, come home and using one of the many methods and oils or formulas in this book, go to bed and make love.

And I mean *make* love – with your eyes, hands, kisses and anything else you can think of.

You could even stay at home in the evening – but make it special. Put the lights down low, play some sensual music and put a few drops of essential oil on a lightbulb. If your partner is willing, you can even watch TV and ask them to gently ease your tension by massaging your shoulders using an essential massage oil.

Choose the oils for your romantic day from the previous list or use one of the formulas below.

Four Sexual Vibration Bath or Shower Formulas

Sandalwood	5 drops	◇	Cypress	3 drops
Geranium	1 drop		Cumin	2 drops
Ylang-ylang	1 drop	◇	Bergamot	2 drops
Nutmeg	2 drops		Rose Maroc	1 drop

The following massage formulas need to be diluted in a dessertspoon of vegetable oil and should be used by both partners on each other.

Three Sexual Vibration Body Massage Formulas

Bergamot	3 drops	Orange	2 drops		Geranium	3 drops
Rose Maroc	2 drops	◇ Rosemary	3 drops	◇	Verbena	2 drops
Cedarwood	1 drop	Ylang-ylang	1 drop		Sandalwood	1 drop

Just turning on the evening news is enough to make even the strongest heart anxious! We live in times of great social tension, and stress has become a way of life. With all there is to worry about, it's no wonder that the real, profound enjoyment of sex can be lost. Sex is, of course, a great stress-reliever – for a few moments everything can be forgotten except emotional feeling and erotic sensation, and then the 'ultimate relief' of orgasm. But using orgasm as a safety valve for pressure somewhat defeats the purpose – to celebrate love with contentment, satisfaction and sublime inexplicable joy. To cross over from 'safety valve' to 'celebration' sex, we need to deal with stress and tension *before* we make love.

In the quiet of therapy rooms, skilled practitioners rebalance the body–mind, bringing harmony with carefully blended oils. All worries go flying out of the window and the patient goes back to work or play better able to deal with problems and enjoy their life.

Male Oils for Stress and Tension

Male Oils for Anxiety

Neroli	Vetiver		Basil	Lavender
Patchouli	Jasmine	◇	Melissa	Coriander
Marjoram	Cedarwood		Ginger	Bergamot

You can use one essential oil alone, or blend the oils of your choice and put them in a small bottle or phial and inhale whenever needed. I know many executives of large companies who wouldn't be without their little bottles in their pockets to help them get through busy days of boardroom meetings, and you'd be surprised to know how many vital decisions on worldwide matters are made with the help of nature's essential oils. Remember that the olfactory cells are technically brain cells and so the molecules go straight where they're needed, to the centre of your motivation and emotion centres, unlike chemical tranquillizers which have to pass through the physical body via the digestive system, bloodstream and then try to get through the blood–brain barrier.

Synergistic Blend
Formulas for Male Anxiety, Stress and Tension

Vetiver	1 drop		Coriander	2 drops
Bergamot	2 drops	◇	Jasmine	1 drop
Geranium	2 drops		Bergamot	2 drops

Neroli	2 drops		Patchouli	1 drop
Lavender	2 drops	◇	Basil	2 drops
Melissa	1 drop		Ginger	2 drops

Basil relaxes the nervous system and also stimulates concentration. Basil has long been used for a clearer, sharper perspective on things, and if you like you can add a drop of basil to the three formulas above which do not already contain it.

If you find the smell of the oils or the formulas too strong in their undiluted form, simply add the proportions above to one teaspoon of pure alcohol, or vodka, or vegetable oil, to make aftershave or body-oil blends. Feel free to make a formula to your own liking from the oils on the lists. They all work as well as each other so it really is a matter of personal preference.

Baths are another very simple method of using nature's oils and are one of the most pleasant ways to release tension from the body and mind. Lie back and encourage the water to lap over your body, letting your cares ease away while concentrating your attention on the aroma of the essential oil. Add a total of four drops, choosing from the lists on page 185 or using one of the suggested formulas below.

Three Baths for Male Stress and Tension

Cedarwood	2 drops		Vetiver	2 drops		Coriander	2 drops
Bergamot	2 drops	◇	Lavender	2 drops	◇	Neroli	2 drops

187

The essential oils are terrific in massages, especially when they're done by another person. As well as the benefits of the molecules entering your system through inhalation and dermis, you get the chance to stay still for a few minutes and enjoy the healing touch of loving hands. But, whether the massage is done by helping hands, or by yourself, rub the oil all over your body paying special attention to the area known as the solar plexus (a round area above your navel), the neck and shoulders. Avoid the genitals. Take your time doing this – don't rush. Choose from the essential oils on page 186, any single or combination up to a total of four drops to a tablespoon of vegetable oil, or try one of my formulas below.

Four Body Massage Formulas for Male Anxiety, Stress and Tension

Jasmine ▶	2 drops of each ◀	Marjoram
Bergamot	combination	Ginger
	into	
Melissa ▶	1 tablespoon of ◀	Cedarwood
Vetiver	vegetable oil	Lavender

If mental fatigue banishes sexual fantasy and vibrancy, physical fatigue leaves you without the energy to make love even though the thought appeals to you. Muscular fatigue can occur at any time in a man's life, the result of overworking the muscles for a long period of time. Providing the fatigue isn't due to injury or illness and you've been diagnosed as fit and healthy except for tiredness, include essential oils in massage and invigorating showers. Nothing works better on a tired body.

This isn't the time to take long, lingering baths, because they only sap your energy more. Save the baths for stress. What you need for muscular fatigue is stimulation by showers, sponging or massage of the muscles. Using the oils mentioned below, add a total of

188

four drops to a sponge or face-cloth in the shower. Don't worry about the essential oil disappearing into the sponge or face-cloth, you'll still get enough benefit using the quantity in this way. Use the oil regularly, every day for two weeks, then rest for one week before continuing treatment again. You'll see that this seemingly small addition to your daily routine will work big wonders!

You can use one or more oils together, to the recommended total of four drops in showers or two in a dessertspoon of vegetable oil for massage. Rosemary is very beneficial on its own for fatigued muscles. Lavender is strengthening. Sage and thyme can ease soreness after exercise. Cypress is excellent for the fibres of the muscles and increases circulation. Eucalyptus stimulates while reducing inflammation. Any combination can help in fatigue.

You can massage your muscles yourself or request the help of your partner or physical therapist. Use any of the oils mentioned above in the same way that a woman would use a body lotion, or copy the suggested combinations below – to a total of two drops of essential oil to one dessertspoon of vegetable oil.

Three Muscular Fatigue Body Massage Oil Formulas

| Rosemary | 1 drop | Cypress | 1 drop | Sage | 1 drop |
| Lavender | 1 drop | Thyme | 1 drop | Eucalyptus | 1 drop |

In a woman the onset of her later years is clearly defined by the menopause. It's often thought that because the male has no such obvious signs of 'the change', and because he can continue to father children long into his old age, that no male menopause exists. From a physical point of view, his 'change' manifests as a gradual reduction in androgen metabolism, but the changes related to this aren't as obvious, or as important from a sexual point of view, as psychological changes which occur around the mid-fifties.

One friend described it to me thus: 'One minute you're thirty, then all of a sudden you're forty and by the time you reach fifty you find yourself saying "when I was a young man . . .", and you realize that you've arrived at old age.' Although still physically strong in his fifties, a man must come to terms with the fact that he is no longer as agile as he was. He can find himself too old for team sports like football, or excusing a bad performance at tennis, for example, by saying, 'If I was my competitor's age I would have won'. Suddenly the doctor is saying, 'It's your age, Mr Jones', and one way and another, a man must confront constant comparison with his youth and the fact that he is growing older. But perhaps the most important difference between a man's youth and later years is in terms of hope, expectation and reality. Old age can be full of disappointments – time is running out and the hope to have been a millionaire by forty has been well and truly worn away by the realization that life is a battle and one is lucky to reach fifty without having a heart-attack or nervous breakdown!

A man in his later years shouldn't waste time pondering on what could have been, but on what is. Contentment is perhaps difficult to achieve simply because the tyranny of the 'winners and losers' syndrome never seems to let up, but it is a wise man – and wisdom comes with age – who recognizes that it's not what a man has that's important, but what a man *is*. Age offers not only liberation in terms of societal pressure to amass material wealth, but also liberation from the idea that the more often one makes love the better, and it can present a man with the opportunity to explore his sexuality as never before. Sexual satisfaction cannot be measured in terms of ejaculation – many men perfunctorily 'perform' the expected deed with little satisfaction for years on end, while many others have sex once a month and experience in that one event a dimension the other men do not yet know. Go for quality rather than quantity.

Read the section 'The masterly stroke' and try to

190

recondition your lovemaking pattern from youth's rushed, excited thrust to ejaculation, to a slower, more prolonged lovemaking pattern. You don't need the great physical energy of youth to be a good lover, and your latter years could provide exactly the incentive you've needed to reassess your sexuality. After all, the inability to achieve immediate subsequent erection/ejaculation does not necessarily equate with a diminished ability to maintain the erection you do have right now. If you think of your later years as a new beginning you may find that the new, concentrated effort to delay ejaculation (and the refractory period) provides you with a chance to explore the potential of experiencing orgasm without ejaculation – a very real physical ability many men never take the time to explore, simply because they've never had the incentive, because they think, 'Well, I can do the whole thing again soon, so why bother to try for multiple orgasms?'.

But if you feel that the mounting pressure of age is being transferred to your lovemaking right now, here are some oils and formulas for you. They will help your body to relax while they stimulate your mind. Use four to six drops in the bath every day for nine days, or in one of the methods of use around the house. You'll be surprised to find how simple it is to regain your confidence while bringing a clarity to your mind. I'm sure you'll find them a wonderful addition to your daily routine.

The Prime Time Oils

Bergamot
Geranium
Cypress
Lavender
Clary-sage
Basil (use half quantities)

Here are three exclusive formulas which will help you both physically and psychologically to regain the energy and optimism of youth. They are synergistic blends, so make up a concentrate and use four drops in a bath or room diffuser. They can also be used very effectively in a water spray or water bowl around the house.

Three Prime Time Synergistic Blends

Bergamot	8 drops	Clary-sage	6 drops	Cypress	8 drops
Lavender	5 drops ◇	Geranium	5 drops ◇	Bergamot	5 drops
Basil	3 drops	Bergamot	6 drops	Clary-sage	4 drops

As far as the TV advertisers are concerned, 'prime time' means peak time for viewing and cashing in. For Aromantics, let prime time be the peak time for living and cashing in on experience, wisdom and love.

THE ASCENT OF MAN

It is a paradox of the male situation that, despite ideas that men 'should be in control' or that 'women are the intuitive ones', that primary symbol of maleness – the penis – is so difficult to control and, more than any other organ of human physiology, so obviously intuitive. Living with this paradox can be very difficult for a man to accept, let alone admit to another person.

Mr E. was forty-four when he came to see me for a back condition that had been extremely painful for a number of years and was getting worse. On examination I found that the whole of his back was in contraction and soon discovered that Mr E. had a very uptight, explosive temperament. Running the course of his treatment he assured me that everything was fine, he had no problems, work was going well, he was successful making new friends, especially women, and there could be no possible underlying cause for the tension which had clearly manifested itself in his back muscles. Things weren't improving as I would expect and so I decided to refer him on. It was at this point that Mr E. decided to reveal his problem – he couldn't get an erection. Very occasionally he could manage a half-erection but that would subside as soon as he tried to penetrate his partner. In effect, penetration was impossible.

Mr E. is typical of many men. He was presenting a very dynamic, 'manly' appearance to the world and literally taking all his stress not only 'on to his shoulders' but all the way down his back and into his sexual life as well. Because Mr E. was so very good at coping on the outside, he found it difficult to accept and admit that he had incorporated stress into his body.

Now that I had the whole picture I formulated a new blend of oils for him and his ladyfriend to use at home and, as his tension eased with the use of the essential oils, so did his erection problem. Because Mr E. had let the situation continue for so long before seeking treatment, it took two months for him to recover his sexuality and longer before the damage in his back muscles could be repaired.

Aggravating and exasperating as loss of erection can be, it may in fact be your body saying 'help'. Never be shy about discussing your sexual vibrancy as a symptom with your doctor – it could give him a vital clue. Many very vague symptoms can seem almost too trivial to discuss and yet can be very important signs of ill-health. Weight loss, indigestion, nausea, stomach ache, tiredness and dizziness, as well as impotence, can be symptoms of many illnesses. Erection difficulties or inability aren't just 'psychological problems' of which you may feel you should be ashamed. If you used to have morning erections and now don't, this could be a sign of diabetes, blocked artery problems, multiple sclerosis, spinal lesions and many other things. Please, don't ignore this sign, saying 'I'm just tired', or excuse it with 'I don't find her attractive any more', or any other excuse – get down to your doctor and insist upon a thorough check-up. Body awareness can save your life. One thing which you cannot help but be aware of is priapism – persistent erection. This is a rare problem, but it could be a hormone imbalance or an enlarged prostate gland causing pressure. Again, down to the doctor straight away.

Many men have suffered their impotence quite alone. Men don't generally exchange information about health and sex, as women do, perhaps because 'locker room' exaggeration doesn't encourage frankness. Some men are reluctant to see the doctor because they think he'll just refer them on to a psychiatrist. In fact, many cases of impotence can be cured quite easily – in the case of venous leak, for example, which is when the blood goes right through the veins of the penis without stopping because the valves don't block off. A minor surgical operation can restore this very easily.

It may also be worth having a discussion with your doctor if you have been prescribed drugs. Sedative, hypnotic drugs like diazepam (Valium) can interfere with libido, as can barbiturates – which can also affect erection and orgasm; chlordiazepoxide (Librium) also affects ejaculation. Some anticholinergic medications used to release bowel spasms can cause impotence and ejaculatory dysfunction, so if you're taking atropine, homatropine, belladonna alkalouds or scopantheline (probanthine) it may be worth considering these as a possible cause of your sexual problems. Even certain nasal decongestants and non-prescription cold remedies containing a combination of antihistamine and anticholinergic drugs may impair libido, erection and ejaculation if taken in doses higher than recommended. You should also be aware that chemical drugs leave a residue in the body and it can take the body some time after cessation of drug treatment to restore harmony.

In fact, when you add up all the possible causes of low sexual vibrancy and response it's a wonder the 'ascent' of man happens at all! All too often the fun of sex turns into the fear of performance, and it's very easy for a minor case of impotence to plummet into a chronic

194

case simply because the man fears a repeat non-performance. Turning to drink at this point is merely going to exacerbate the problem, so don't bother with that. Instead, turn to your bottles of essential oils, because they do infinitely more good.

Don't expect the essential oils to work immediately like the 'super-stud' preparations you can buy in sex shops are supposed to (they don't have the best reputation anyway). Nature likes to take her time. It may take you just a couple of applications, it may take a couple of months, but the results will be well worth waiting for. Anything that promises immediate erection is likely to be dangerous. Probably the best-known male aphrodisiac is 'Spanish fly' – the beetle which contains a poison, cantharides, which has properties that cause irritation of the penis and whole urinary system including erection. If taken internally Spanish fly can cause innumerable problems which, according to Herbert Seymour, end in 'perforation of the stomach, ulcers throughout the entire length of the intestinal canal, dysentery and lastly death in the midst of intolerable agonies'. Obviously, a so-called aphrodisiac to be avoided at all costs! Despite its dreadful reputation, Spanish fly seems to have gone down in folklore as the ultimate aphrodisiac and this just proves how desperate men have been to improve their performance. Indeed, some of the preparations on record are very convoluted to prepare, bizarre to imagine and dangerous to use. In an extremely amusing account by a 'French Army Surgeon' of his explorations into the sexual customs of people in various far-flung corners of the world in the 1860s to 1890s, he records a method used in Guyana, South America, called 'tightening wood' – made from the bark of a local tree, 'to make him perform often'. This same ingredient is included with seven other ingredients (including phosphorous matches!) in a paste which is encased with the erect penis in the skin of a hollowed-out aubergine (egg-plant) 'of an appropriate size'. After a couple of minutes this produces 'intense' inflammation of the penis so it needs to be bathed in yet another concoction. The 'copulation' is said to be 'almost painful'. I bet! If you think that sounded difficult, try this advice from the *Kama Sutra*: 'First rub your penis with wasp stings and massage it with sweet oil. When it swells, let it dangle for ten nights through a hole in your bed, going to sleep each night on your stomach.'

But enough of this nonsense, let's take a look at the list of harmless yet effective essential oils which can be used for erection difficulties and impotence.

Essential Oils to Help with Erection Difficulties

Ambrette	Ginger
Anis vert	Lavender
Anis	Mace
Basil	Orange
Clove	Rose Maroc
Clary-sage	Rosemary
Coriander	Sage
Celery	Savory
Cinnamon	Sandalwood
Fenugreek	Thyme

Men have been using these substances for centuries to improve the hardness and duration of their erection. Don't make up your own mixtures from these oils – either select one to use on its own or follow one of my formulas. We shall be looking at three different types of erection difficulty, each with its own formulas, so try to identify the situation that seems best suited to you.

We begin with the formulas for erection difficulties related to anxiety, stress and tension, and these are usually easily sorted out. You can do the treatment on your own, but if you have a partner it's preferable for them to join you. Although erection difficulties can make the sufferer feel very alone in the world, it's often forgotten that the partner can feel responsible in some way, and inadequate because they cannot induce an erection – they can feel just as alone. Use this time to allow the partner to express their compassion and understanding and as a time of coming back together.

Start the treatment by massaging your partner (if your partner is male, he should try to refrain from getting an erection himself at this point because that will only exacerbate your feelings of inadequacy). Massage your partner's back in a slow and relaxed way. As the molecules of essential oil will be seeping into your own system via the sense of smell, mixing now with your partner's pheromones, inhale deeply and experience the erotic mix of aromas. If you're using the correct blend, you – the masseur – will find yourself becoming calm and relaxed too. The essential oils have a soothing effect on the central nervous system and, contrary to popular belief, a calm and relaxed nervous system responds sexually much more readily than an overanxious one. For this massage oil, choose a combination of any three essential oils from the list below, added to vegetable oil.

The Sexy, Relaxing Body Massage Oils

Lemon	Cumin	Coriander	Sandalwood
Geranium	Clary-sage	Rose Maroc	

Here are some tried and tested formulas. You can both use these synergistic blends except for one small, but important, difference – the man with the erection difficulty uses the blend with one drop of ginger.

For your Partner and Yourself,
Four Sexy, Relaxing Synergistic Blends

Clary-sage	5 drops	For your partner	Cumin	5 drops
Rose Maroc	5 drops ▶	Make a concentrate	◀ Geranium	5 drops
Sandalwood	5 drops	using these proportions,	Clary-sage	5 drops
		then put 4 drops of		
Coriander	5 drops	concentrate into 1	Rose Maroc	5 drops
Geranium	5 drops ▶	teaspoon of	◀ Coriander	5 drops
Lemon	5 drops	vegetable oil	Lemon	5 drops

For you
As above, but add 1 drop of ginger

When it is the turn of the man with the erection difficulty to be massaged, his partner should pay special attention to the area of the lower back two inches above the waist down to the crease of the buttocks, but making sure to avoid the anus.

If you don't have a partner right now, or if you don't want your partner to play a part in this treatment, massage yourself using the formula below. Massage your solar plexus with one hand, rubbing in circles in an anticlockwise direction until you feel a sense of relaxation. Then move to the lower back area just mentioned. Do this massage daily for nine days preparatory to seeing your lover, including the day of your date.

The 'On-Your-Own' Erection Formula

Cumin	2 drops
Ginger	2 drops
Black pepper	2 drops
Anise	2 drops

In 1 dessertspoon of vegetable oil

Clearly, massage of the lower back is easier done by a helping hand, although it's perfectly possible to do it yourself if you want to keep this treatment private. If you do have a lover who can join in, you'll both benefit by inhaling the essential oils, so just enjoy touching each other without any performance pressure. Be patient, and remember, if at first you don't succeed . . .

Next we come to the formula for the man with a slightly different problem. This is characterized by a normal sexual appetite, erotic fantasies and a strong desire to make love – but weak erection. It's an extremely frustrating form of erection difficulty because the urge, interest and desire are there, but not the ability. Often this is related to drug or alcohol use, loss of confidence or other psychological problems which have led to nervous tension. Many different groups of men may be encompassed here; for example, those who feel guilty, perhaps for extra-marital affairs, and find that they cannot make love with their wife, although they may still be quite capable of producing an erection with another woman. Sometimes the problem stems from a bout of boredom setting a pattern of non-erection which cannot now be lost.

This situation can be equally frustrating for both partners. It's important at this time to avoid trying to penetrate when the erection isn't really ready yet – that only exacerbates the exasperation! Don't think lovemaking has to come to a disastrous end just because your penis isn't ready and able. Forget about your penis for a while (it'll be ready soon enough) and spend this interim time exploring the possibilities of non-penile sex.

Here then is the formula for men with strong sexual desire but a weak erection. Apply the massage formula once a day for two weeks and then follow up with the formula(s) that seem to suit you best from the 'Releasing your sexual vibration' section (page 185). Massage the lower back down just into the crease of the buttocks but not as far as the anus, and also on the upper thighs but avoiding (and I mean avoiding) the genitals. Regular use of the following formula will produce a stronger and longer erection – and I mean by the clock, not the centimetre.

The Stronger, Longer Erection Formula

Ginger	*2 drops*
Black pepper	*2 drops*
Savory	*2 drops*

In 1 tablespoon of vegetable oil

Now we come to the two-part, nine-day treatment for men who have been given a clean bill of health by their doctor and yet who have suffered a long period of erection difficulty. This is the super-resuscitation formula that will bring vibrant life back to any man who has been worn down by any one of the many causes of male impotence.

The Super Rooster Booster

Days 1–4 *Mix equal proportions in a clean bottle then use ▶ 3 drops each day on a sponge and rub over the whole body*

Synergistic blend
Savory
Rosemary
Peppermint
Neroli

Days 5–9 *Mix, then add the total 8 drops to a sitz bath and ▶ relax for 3–5 minutes*

Savory	*2 drops*
Peppermint	*2 drops*
Lavender	*2 drops*
Thyme	*1 drop*
Rosemary	*1 drop*

Of course, as any man who has made it to the top will tell you, getting there is only half the battle – staying in position is another problem! Premature ejaculation is a very widespread problem in our culture, partly due to the fact that men have masturbated with a feeling of shame when growing up, and got into the habit of ejaculating quickly, before they get caught. This 'rapid-fire' situation gets transferred to lovemaking later on. Young men suffer premature ejaculation when starting out because of over-excitement, and many men of all ages suffer it at the onset of new relationships. Older men can find that they suffer premature ejaculation more frequently, as can men who have sex infrequently or men who visit prostitutes, who always have one eye on the clock.

The anxiety of being unable to maintain an erection for as long as a man would like is something which has to be treated before anything else, because the idea of failure is a self-fulfilling prophecy. Rub this formula over the abdomen before having sex.

The 'Holding Back' Body Massage Formula

Clary-sage	1 drop
Nutmeg	1 drop
Vetiver	1 drop

Into 1 teaspoon of vegetable oil

When you make love, incorporate the Masters and Johnson 'squeeze' technique into your lovemaking routine. (You can practise this on your own, following as best you can the directions for the woman's hand positions.) The woman sits opposite the man, perhaps with her back resting against something, and the man lies with his legs over her hips. Her thumb rests against the frenulum, the triangular-shaped membrane where the shaft joins the ridge on the underside of the penis: her index finger curls around and rests on the glans, above the ridge; and her middle finger is just below the ridge, so that her fingers have this ridge between them. When she applies the 'squeeze', the woman presses between thumb and two fingers for about four seconds. The urge to ejaculate is lost and, after about fifteen to thirty seconds, on his signal, she can begin the stimulation again. The squeeze technique can easily be incorporated into intercourse in the female-superior and side-by-side positions. When you feel as if you're about to ejaculate, separate your body from hers and let her apply the squeeze. Do this at least five times before allowing yourself to ejaculate and if you get a bit soft, she can revive you or you can revive yourself. Timing is everything in the squeeze. If you're practising on your own, however, you can keep a tighter control. Approach ejaculation progressively, on tiptoe so to speak, not going too close to ejaculation on the run up to the first couple of squeezes.

All the while you're making love, inhale the aroma of the essential oils, which will now be getting warm, allowing the aroma to enter the brain and limbic system. During the proceedings, once more rub the massage oil into the abdomen. Excitement will be high by now and the oils will be producing a relaxed, euphoric atmosphere.

Some men want everything at once and to be cured yesterday, and yet won't want to bother with trying the technique outlined above. What can I say? They might like to try another system – which isn't as effective because its effect will be less on the penis and more on the brain – using one of the oils below in one of the room methods. Any of the oils can also be incorporated into a massage formula of your own making.

Essential Oils that Can Help Combat Premature Ejaculation

Clary-sage	Hyacinth
Nutmeg	Marjoram
Vetiver	Chamomile Maroc
Narcissus	Benzoin

Massage oil: 5 drops per 1 teaspoon of vegetable oil
Room diffusers: 10 drops

Here are some formulas that work well in both massage oil and room diffusers. Use every day for at least two weeks, especially on the nights when love is in the air.

Four Formulas to Combat Premature Ejaculation

Narcissus	2 drops	◇	Vetiver	2 drops
Nutmeg	2 drops		Chamomile Maroc	2 drops
Marjoram	2 drops	◇	Hyacinth	2 drops
Clary-sage	2 drops		Benzoin	2 drops

Massage oil: dilute in 1 tablespoon of vegetable oil
Room diffusers: double quantity

Experiment with sexual positions and find one in which penile stimulation isn't so great. Understand that you are not alone in the world with this problem. Have patience, use your intuition, and you will find yourself regaining control.

THE MASTERLY STROKE

For a 'liberated' society, we still have enormous guilt about masturbation. The Hite Reports on both male and female sexuality are stuffed with negativity on this subject, and this despite the fact that just about everyone today realizes that masturbation isn't going to get them locked up, or cause blindness, warts, insanity or general physical disintegration! Research shows that men feel guilty, inadequate, defensive and lonely when masturbating; that they do not tell others that they do it; and feel that it's only justified as a substitute for 'the real thing'.

The problems start when the precocious sexuality of children gets slapped down by parents who, quite understandably, are worried that if little Frank doesn't realize that playing with himself is naughty, whenever he gets bored at kindergarten he'll pull out his penis.

The message comes across early – don't do it! Even under the bedclothes, we're told, God can see what's going on, and the church view has been quite clear: the Vatican has called it 'a seriously disordered act'. I mean, who wants to own up to that?

And yet, the sex urge is there. Kinsey found that boys at puberty weren't unusual if they masturbated half a dozen times a day and as young people have so little privacy, no doubt that masturbation was guilty and rushed, while looking over the shoulder.

How much better it would be to teach a boy that masturbation is a natural part of growing up and, therefore, something to be enjoyed, taking as much pleasure from it as possible and as much time as necessary to prolong the sensation, in readiness for the greater sensation of making love. If parents were to do this, premature ejaculation wouldn't be such a problem to their sons, and boys might learn how to separate the two distinct physical processes of what they now understand to be the one – orgasm.

Some societies knew, thousands of years before Masters and Johnson 'discovered' in the West, that the male sexual response pattern is actually composed of two quite separate physical processes – orgasm and ejaculation – and have encouraged men into training so that they can enjoy prolonged lovemaking routines, not only for the benefit of their partner, but for the benefit of themselves. In different societies, the understanding of male sexuality has taken varied routes because of differing philosophies. In India, sex is very much involved with spiritual development, not only because one of the four aims of Hindu life is to enjoy sensual and sexual pleasure – rejoice in life's beauty – but also because in channelling sexual energy correctly through chakras (energy centres), the so-called supernatural faculties could be developed. In China, the emphasis was on sex as medicine and very much concerned with prolonged lovemaking, because then the man could absorb through the membranes of his penis the chemicals in the female sexual juices – adding 'yin' to his 'yang' and creating 'ch'i', the vital force which rejuvenates the body and mind. Indeed, longevity was thought to depend upon a good sex life and, specifically, non-ejaculation after prolonged lovemaking during which the man, as well as the woman, would enjoy many orgasms.

It would take a whole book to go into the routines which other cultures have developed to facilitate male orgasm while avoiding ejaculation, so here I will have to concentrate on the most important areas and the use of nature's oils.

The first area to develop for good ejaculatory control is your breathing patterns. Breathing is something we usually take no notice of, but it does vary. Before a job interview you may take a couple of deep breaths, and if you're trying to overhear a conversation you may stop breathing momentarily to aid concentration. There is a correlation between the motion of breath and the motion of a man's ejaculatory process – if you can control your breathing pattern, you can control the path of your semen, too. As you approach orgasm, breathing gets racy and out of control. The breaths are shallow, involving just the top of the lung, possibly taken through an open mouth – more of a pant than a breath. Strained, shallow breathing makes the semen speed up on its course while deep, rhythmic breathing slows it down; and temporary arrest of breath, in conjunction with other methods, brings it to a halt.

For controlled and prolonged lovemaking, your breath should be taken through the nose and right down to the lower abdomen, gently and rhythmically. This counteracts the sympathetic nervous system, which produces the adrenaline which in turn triggers ejaculation. When you feel yourself getting carried away, switch your attention immediately to the pattern of your breathing. Concentrate on the fact that your lungs are inflating and deflating, be aware that your chest is moving up and down and the air is going through the nostrils. Lock your attention into these physical processes and block out of your conciousness physical processes going on elsewhere. Whatever you do, do not think about your penis! Or your orgasm! If you allow such thoughts into your imagination you'll get carried away and indeed have that orgasm. Again, while locking yourself into the pattern of your breathing, cease all movement. You should try to adopt this breath-consciousness while masturbating; and when lovemaking, at the point of crisis ask your partner to stop all movement, too.

Because masturbation is so often excused as a sort of toiletry habit and referred to as 'relieving tension', I think it's best to set aside a particular time, preplanned, rather than merely masturbate as the result of the 'immediate urge'. The fact of preplanning implies a respectful taking of responsibility. Look forward to your special time, take the phone off the hook and prepare your oils!

First, a word of warning. When I say one drop, *use only one drop* and not two or three, or you'll end up with an irritant reaction like Spanish fly instead of a soothing, pleasurable sensation.

So, in a liqueur glass, which is roughly one ounce, pour in your base-oil. The best to use here is almond oil which is nice and light and, as a bonus, nourishes the skin. Add a total of three drops of essential oil only, choosing from the erogenous oils below.

The Masterly Stroke Training Oils

Cumin	Patchouli	Ylang-ylang
Coriander	Sandalwood	Tonka bean
Jasmine	Rose Maroc	Cardamom
Nutmeg	Ambrette	

Try blending a combination of two or three oils on the list – your preference is all-important. Below are some suggested combinations you may like to try.

Four Masterly Stroke Training Formulas

Rose Maroc	1 drop		Jasmine	1 drop
Cumin	1 drop	◇	Ambrette	1 drop
Tonka bean	1 drop		Coriander	1 drop

Ylang-ylang	1 drop		Nutmeg	1 drop
Sandalwood	1 drop	◇	Rose Maroc	1 drop
Cardamom	1 drop		Patchouli	1 drop

Add to 30 ml of almond oil

When you've made up your formula, apply a little of the oil to the lower abdomen, just above the pubic hair. This is a particularly sensitive area which responds well to slight pressure and when rubbed gently and rhythmically in a circular, clockwise movement can produce an erection fairly easily. (If you have a partner handy, she can massage you to erection by rubbing a band about four inches high, on either side of the vertebrae at the base of your spine.) Explore the sensitivity of your upper thighs and scrotum. Take your time and enjoy the sensation of being erect for a while.

Now gently stimulate the shaft of your penis, smoothing the oil up in whichever way you desire. Explore the special sensitivity of the frenulum, the little triangular piece of membrane just under the coronal ridge. Feel the different sensations you can elicit during this time at the head or base of the penis, along the vein on the underside, the inner thigh – wherever and all over. Soon enough you'll begin to feel like stimulating yourself to orgasm and OK, carry on, but before you feel the point of no return approaching, *stop*. What is your breath doing now – it's rapid, isn't it? So slow it down. Close your eyes, take your hand away, breathe deeply and rhythmically through the nose until you regain your composure. Now, start the stimulation again. When you feel orgasm approaching, *stop*.

If things are getting unbearable, try squeezing as described for the technique on page 201. You could also try another technique much admired in the East – with the middle finger of your free hand press firmly into the spot midway between your scrotum and anus. This is an acupressure point which stops the passage of semen. By the way, don't worry about what will happen if you play around like this and don't ejaculate – the seminal fluid gets taken into the bladder and is flushed out through the penis with your next urination. Men have been doing this for centuries with no recorded ill-effects.

This type of manual training technique combined with breathing awareness will, if performed regularly, bring ejaculation under your control. When you're ready to transfer to sexual intercourse, it will allow you the opportunity to concentrate on your sensations, which is important because the ultimate goal is to be able to identify the approach to, and actual moment in, the male orgasmic experience when the orgasm and ejaculation are separated, usually by a second or two. That second or two can be extended so that you can experience the orgasm, or orgasms, while keeping ejaculation at bay. This is super-ejaculation control!

Once you have the masterly stroke you'll be released from the tyranny of fear that comes with being unable to hold back, and free to allow your woman really to express herself sexually. Don't just use your new-found ejaculation control to extend the time you impose your sexual rhythm on her – she has a rhythm, too, and it may not be the same as yours. We're so used to the idea that women 'respond' to the male rhythm, that many women have no idea what their own rhythm is (except when they masturbate alone). Stay still for a while and say to her, 'You move to your own rhythm, don't worry about me'. After all, think about it, your orgasm is dependent upon you being able to move freely in a precise rhythm, so why shouldn't rhythm be as important to her? Now's your chance to liberate both of you, and you can both enjoy each other's rhythms, build up the passion and reach new heights!

BODY AWARENESS

Body awareness doesn't take much, but it can save a lot! If you saw the movie *Champions*, you'll already know how important it is to go to your doctor if you have a swollen testicle. Top jockey Bob Champion had a slightly numb, painless, swollen testicle for about three months before he was lucky enough to find himself in bed with an American lady vet who knew how dangerous this sign was and made him promise to contact his doctor as soon as he returned home, the next day.

At the airport, Bob phoned his doctor and within hours was having tests. Twenty-four hours later, he had an operation to remove one testicle. Bob Champion was lucky. If he'd continued to ignore the swelling he reckons he would have been dead in about eight months. Instead, he went on to win the Grand National and father his baby son, Michael.

Testicular cancer is the commonest cancer in young men and it's on the increase. At the moment, one in five hundred British men under forty-five will be affected, but by the year 2000 doctors fear that the numbers will be closer to one in every two hundred men. Since 1961 the figures have gone up 80 per cent for men between the ages of twenty-five and thirty-four. Early diagnosis is the difference, if not between life and death exactly (with the present 90 per cent cure rate), then between easy and difficult treatment. The ones who die are the ones who went to their doctors months, sometimes years, after they'd noticed the first symptoms. The problem seems to be that either the men are embarrassed about the idea of a problem 'down there': they mistake the increased size of the testicle as improved virility; or, simply, they never touch themselves around the testicles and hadn't noticed any change.

Men are advised to check once a month while lying in a hot bath, while the supporting muscles are relaxed. Roll the testicles individually between the thumbs and fingers of both hands feeling for any tenderness, numbness, hard lumps or nodules. Watch out for any swelling, which could be general and painless, or small, hard nodules which can be distinguished from the normal consistency of the testicles. This could be a tumour and it can grow quickly, doubling in size every three weeks or so. The two testicles often vary in size and that is perfectly normal, but their consistency should feel about the same. Back pain is another symptom, as is any dull ache in the lower abdomen and groin. Men who have had a testicle which didn't drop into the scrotal pouch are ten times more likely to develop testicular cancer and must obviously make a special note.

If you see any changes in your body that look as if they shouldn't be there (and I'm not talking about flab!), get along to your medical practitioner without delay. It is better to be safe than sorry. Explain all your symptoms, even the seemingly unimportant ones that came and went some time ago. In Europe, the medicinal school which uses nature's essential oils is known as phytotherapy, and hundreds of doctors of medicine choose to specialize in it, recognizing not only that the essential oils provide effective and safer alternatives to modern drugs, but that they can be used in all medical conditions. The medicinal scope of nature's essential oils spans from the oldest and most mundane human ailment – broken bones which ginger encourages to heal – to the most modern and dangerous, HIV, which the Pasteur Institute, amongst others, is trying to fight by extending their antiviral weaponry.

6

The Other Side

Sex has always had a difficult and dangerous side. In 1903, 41 per cent of the recruits from Berlin applying to join the Prussian Army were rejected for having syphilis – and in 1903 syphilis was a killer. Today we're terrified of being told that we are HIV positive, but there is more to worry about than that.

Cervical cancer is known to be more likely if the woman has been in sexual contact with a partner with genital warts. We don't think of human papilloma virus (HPV) as a killer, but HPV can be a crucial co-factor in the development of cancerous cells, and it's thought, to a lesser degree, that herpes simplex can be too. The BMA estimate that a woman having sex with a man with genital warts has a one in three chance of developing a pre-cancerous condition of the cervix. Another very dangerous sexually transmitted disease is chlamydia, which can infect the Fallopian tubes and cause a blockage so that an ectopic pregnancy occurs. Like many sexually transmitted diseases, chlamydia can be completely symptomless. More often than not, men and women pass each other life-long problems in complete innocence. This has been very much the case with AIDS.

When we talk about sexually transmitted diseases we're actually talking about a whole variety of viruses, bacteria, fungi, yeasts and protozoa. The diseases these little invaders cause include AIDS, herpes, genital warts, syphilis, gonorrhoea, chlamydia, gardnerella, trichomonas, thrush and non-specific infections. All these problems affect both men and women, either of whom can be symptomless.

There are many reasons for people to regret having a particular sexual liaison, but because partners usually pass the problems on unknowingly, laying blame is unnecessary and unhelpful. It's very unfortunate, but sexually transmitted diseases can happen to anyone. We need to be aware of the problems rather than try to pretend that they don't happen . . . and certainly not to us. The only way to be certain is to go for regular check-ups at the local specialist clinic, and immediately if there are any unusual signs of disease because herpes, for example, can only be identified when there are physical signs on the body. Becoming aware and responsible about sexual hazards is our best line of defence against them. We owe this not only to ourselves and our present and future partners but to all our unborn children, the very existence of whom may depend upon our sexual health.

The condom is an excellent line of defence, especially when lubricated with *nonoxynol-9* spermicide, but it doesn't seem to be everyone's favourite item. We've all heard that using condoms is like 'wearing wellingtons in the bath', or 'eating chocolate with the wrapper on', and it is this unerotic aspect that causes nations to shun responsibility for inventing it – the French call it the 'English hood', while the English call it the 'French letter'! However, whatever the condom's disadvantages, it remains the best immediate protection against all sexually transmitted diseases, and for those not in a monogamous relationship condoms are clearly a vital item to have in the bathroom cabinet or bedside table.

Reluctant condom-users must constantly remind themselves that the vast majority of HIV carriers look and feel perfectly healthy because the virus can take years to develop. These days it is best to play safe; and the safer the better. Caution and precaution are the order of the day, and to this, nature's essential oils can add a much-needed note of eroticism.

WHAT'S THE FIVE-LETTER WORD THAT TOOK THE 'S' OUT OF SEX?

V-I-R-U-S. First it was the virus herpes, now it's HIV, which causes AIDS, and the virus which causes genital warts has been coming and going all along.

'V' is for vampire, which is what a virus is. It inhabits a strange world of limbo between death and life, itself technically unalive because it can't move, act or reproduce on its own. A virus only comes alive when it has invaded living matter – bacteria, plants, animals or human beings. This 'host' provides the very life-force of the virus through whichever 'host-cell' each type of virus takes over.

'I' is for the immune system, the body's self-defence mechanisms. This has two armies: firstly, the white blood cells which cruise around the blood and lymph streams, engulfing bacteria and other alien invaders and escorting them out through the exits – urine, faeces and perspiration. Secondly, we have antibodies – 'instant' armies produced specifically to deal with a particular type of invader. Antibodies are produced in the spleen and lymph nodes with locate-and-destroy mechanisms tailor-made for each type of incoming invader. Immunity against a particular disease means that your body has already taken a pattern of the antibodies it will need to produce if and when that particular alien invades again, and so will deal more effectively with it.

'R' is for the retrovirus HIV, which is so darn clever it's threatening the 'U' and the 'S' – us! This virus chooses for its host-cells T-lymphocytes, white blood cells, and uses the impressive reproductive capacity of

213

the T-cell to transform the genetic information within its protein shell into thousands of clones of itself. In this process the virus clones destroy ever-increasing numbers of T-cells, while also hijacking their reproductive potential. This is what leads to the 'I' and 'D' in AIDS – immune deficiency.

Each day we hear more about the HIV virus and with each revelation it becomes more and more clear that this little monster is dead smart. It can fool the antibodies with its 'antigenic drift' – which means that it can change the structure of its protein shell so that the original pattern or blueprint of the invader no longer fits, and so the antibody just passes HIV by. Because of HIV's now-you-see-me-now-you-don't quality it's going to be very difficult to make a vaccine.

Also, the HIV virus can shed its protein shell so that, even if an antibody manages to recognize and stick to it, the shell just comes off 'in its hands', so to speak. This process has been described as 'analogous to a lizard losing its tail when attacked by a predator',* and is dangerous because the protein shell can then become attached to other cells, and thus direct the body's own antibodies to attack and destroy these cells.

HIV is patient, too. It can hang out for up to fifteen years just being as unobtrusive as possible, hiding or slowly taking over its favourite host-cells – T-lymphocytes. Depending upon the degree of takeover, the host organism – a person affected by HIV – falls prey to serious uncontrolled invasion by the other viruses, protozoa, fungi or bacteria, because the T-cells are too busy to deal with them while they're fighting their own battle with HIV.

To summarize then, HIV infiltrates and destroys one half of the immune system's defending army – the T-cells – while fooling the other half – the antibodies. While all this is going on all manner of other invaders take over the body, usually making the carrier so ill that he or she dies.

*New Scientist, 26 March 1987.

Looking at it this way, it's clear that HIV doesn't win, because when the carrier dies, HIV is thought to die with it. But HIV is patient and all the while has been making clones of itself, which get passed from person to person, on and on, so that if on a small scale the success of HIV is limited, because of its clones, in evolutionary terms HIV is highly successful.

As a society, our best defence against HIV largely depends upon our ability to contain HIV from being passed from 'host' person to person by practising sexual abstinence or safer sex. Enter the condom.

As individuals, our best defence is to have a good, strong immune system. This is one that flows vigorously, providing an efficient invader-and-garbage collection service with lots of white blood cells ready to fight the ever-threatening aliens. Every part of this system, from the free-roaming white blood cells to the cell substance interferon (which stops multiple virus development), needs an adequate supply of amino acids which, because of their metabolism, need vitamins and minerals. These are the nutrients which we need to keep our immune system in peak fighting condition.

Building up our immune system as a deliberate ploy to make ourselves less vulnerable is something everyone should be considering at this difficult time – and if not for reasons of sexual safety, then for general health and as protection against Hong Kong flu or some other viral problem. We're all losing out on 'natural goodness', day by day, in many small but accumulatively important ways. The food we eat is depleted of its nutrients, such as vitamins, minerals and trace elements, because of over-farming, chemical fertilizers, processing, preservatives, irradiation and, very important, long periods of storage. This is just one problem. We breathe lead in with our air and drink fluoride with our water. Living in the concrete jungle builds up positive ions that can have a distressing effect on the body. Some people walk barefoot on grass and earth to help discharge this static electricity.

The subject of vitamins, minerals and trace elements

is too wide and complex to go into here, so I strongly suggest that you extend your knowledge by referring to the many books on the market which discuss diet, especially those for fighting cancer and AIDS. As a brief guide, however, I would recommend you take the following amino acids: glycine, which initiates antibody action; cysteine, which can detoxify and improve healing and builds disease resistance; lysine, a bacterial invasion resistant; phenylalanine, which is important in fighting infection, soothes pain and is said to create an increased energy level; taurine, which cleans out free radicals (scavenger cells thought to be carcinogenic); and glutathione, which helps neutralize and destroy free radicals. Also important for the good health of the immune system are vitamins A, C, E and B-complex and the trace elements selenium and zinc.

As well as redressing nutritional imbalances, we need to consider the need to redress environmental ones. It's been found that people subjected to daily smoke and industrial waste suffer blockages of the lymph nodes near their lungs. Their 'clearage' system cannot deal with the volume of work it is now expected to do. To counteract this, try to get as much fresh air as possible by going for walks in the country. We need the oxygen to keep the blood and lymph systems all flowing along, a process which aids the elimination of toxins. Also, try to get into the sunshine whenever you can – not to tan or burn, just soak in the sun. And if you're really serious, give up smoking and drinking . . . give your body a break!

The immune system is known to be negatively affected by psychological factors, like stress, which is why herpes attacks occur at times of trouble (when they are least needed!). Clearly, the AIDS epidemic provides everyone with the incentive to identify those areas of our lives which are stressful so that we can attempt to deal with them once and for all. Allow yourself to express your emotions – hang what people think. Be yourself and don't keep things pent up inside. Clear the decks of stress and negative emotion and do everything

216

possible to keep life calm and evenly balanced – and get enough sleep. Meditation, yoga and relaxation techniques can also be very helpful.

It now seems clear that some people are less prone to HIV than others and it could be that some people have a built-in immunity to it. It also seems that some people, once infected, develop the symptomatic disease quicker than others – i.e., they are overwhelmed by invading organisms because their T-cells can't deal with them. It seems possible, too, that a configuration of factors can spark off a more serious viral infection, so if you're prone to colds and bouts of flu, or have a history of herpes (or fungal and bacterial infections), you should perhaps take more care now to strengthen your immune system.

In the battle against HIV we need all the help we can get. If it seems strange to turn to nature's essential oils for help, bear in mind that these are the substances that give plants protection against enemy pests, bacteria, viruses and fungi. Leaves ooze their aromatic protection while flowers emit a cloud of airborne particles into their perfumed 'headspace'. The use of nature's oils as an antibacterial agent is quite well known, but they're used, too, against viral invasions by doctors, phytotherapists and other medical practitioners.

Essential oils are now being used by building services managers to clean bacteria and fungi out of air-conditioning systems in large buildings. CIG, part of the multinational BOC, are marketing a product called Bactigas, which is essentially tea-tree oil. A fine mist permeates the air-conditioning system overnight, leaving the air in the building clean and fresh and, as a bonus, invigorating to the people working there. It also reduces the incidence of colds and flu among the workers, and cuts down on the mould and mildew which eats paintwork away. As time progresses we shall undoubtedly see an increased use of essential oils – no manager wants to be responsible for an outbreak of legionnaires' disease in his building. The potential of essential oils for reducing infection in hospitals is simply vast.

217

Nature's essential oils make excellent cleansing agents – anti-toxins. They work through the lymphatic system, aiding the elimination of toxic matter. Stress and anxiety reduce blood and lymph flow, and by alleviating stress the essential oils effectively allow a more vigorous flow so that toxins can be eliminated more efficiently. However, it is extremely important to do this gently, over a period of time, enabling the release of toxins to happen slowly so that no blockages occur in the lymph nodes. I must reiterate this point – slowly and gently clear toxins from the body. The essential oils also have a stimulating and strengthening effect on the lymphatic system as a whole, which means that there are more white blood cells to help fight the ever-incoming invaders. Certain oils also stimulate the regeneration of tissue which can help the cells that got caught in the fray.

At the London Lighthouse, one of the world's foremost centres for treating AIDS, aromatherapy is routinely given to both residential and day-care service users. The reason given for this is that it promotes a state of well-being which is, in itself, an important factor in prolonging health. Research has shown that this 'sense of well-being' is a more crucial element in the development or non-development of opportunistic infection than the number of T-cells present. An average healthy person has about 1000 T-cells while an HIV carrier will not usually be put on AZT until that number has dropped to 200. However, people with counts very much below this still maintain good health if their sense of well-being is good and their attitude positive.

Well-being Formula

Italian everlasting	10 drops
Lemongrass	5 drops
Patchouli	1 drop
Geranium	2 drops
Clove	1 drop
Cinnamon	1 drop
Bergamot	5 drops

Prepare in a 30 ml bottle

The way you prepare this formula is important. Start by mixing the cinnamon, clove, patchouli and lemongrass in your empty 30 ml bottle. Blend these well together. Then add the geranium, Italian everlasting and berga-mot, and blend well again. Now add the base-oil, which should be sweet almond, and blend again.

This formula can be used with a partner or in conjunc-tion with the self-massage techniques on page 101. Do not apply to the face.

Essential oils routinely travel in the bloodstream, lymph flow and interstitial fluid and, unlike chemical drugs, they're completely compatible with the human body, and in their correct dosage they are completely harmless. The ones mentioned here all work in slightly different ways. Oregano, thyme and Italian everlasting are known and used antiviral agents. Italian everlast-ing, as well as being antibacterial, stimulates the lymphatic flow through the kidneys and liver, a process which helps the elimination of toxins. Lavender helps in the reproduction of cells, rebuilding the damage constantly being done because of the virus's *modus operandi*, as well as being antibiotic, anti-venomous and increasing lymphatic flow. Geranium helps the blood circulation, in a general sense aiding the vigour of the blood–lymph system.

I cannot say that essential oils will prevent you catching viruses, but if used properly and carefully they can offer additional protection. Certainly, more research should be done on them in the search for a cure for AIDS. However, in the unsexy age of 'safer sex', the protective essential oils must surely be one of the most pleasant ways to help yourself by adding eroticism to protection. The oils can be used in many different ways but are, perhaps, at their most erotic when used in a massage oil. They are very strong and should be kept away from condoms, which they could possibly break. But a cautious use of both condoms and essential oils, and a concerted effort to attend to the health of our immune system, will together offer a good package of safer sex when caution is required. It's a cliché, but it's true – it's better to be safe than sorry.

The Protective Essential Oils

Antiviral   **Antifungal**

Oregano   *These are*   *Patchouli*   *Some of the*
Thyme   ◄   *among the*   ◄   *Tea tree*   ◄   *best antifungal*
Italian   *most effective*   *Clove*   *oils*
everlasting   *Geranium*
Cinnamon   *Lemongrass*
                                     Palma rosa

Antibacterial

Lavender   *Myrtle*
Balsam de Peru   *Thyme*
Pine   *Oregano*
Niaouli   *Cinnamon*
Bergamot   *Tea tree*
Italian everlasting   *Cedarwood*

**Antiseptic and
disinfectant**
Palma rosa
Lime
Grapefruit
Lemon

Sage   *These are more in harmony with the*
Clary-sage   ◄   *treatment of female problems because*
Rose   *of their hormone-like properties*

Marjoram   ◄   *Not a sexy oil*

Clove   *Aphrodisiacs, but highly irritant in*
Cinnamon   ◄   *large doses*

EXTRA-SAFE SEX

There are several methods you can use to help protect
yourself from the various little organisms that bug us.
In this section I have included a super-protection

221

THE PROTECTIVE ESSENTIAL OILS

Essential oils are often more effective in a synergistic mix but each has protective merits as well as curative ones.

BALSAM DE PERU *(Myroxylon pereirae)* **Antibacterial** **Antiseptic** **Possibly antifungal**	This is not an essential oil as such, but a resinoid or resin obtained from a tree which grows in South America. Although used for coughs and respiratory problems, it has an excellent effect against invading bacteria and infections of the genital tract. Very good as an antiseptic and it has a wonderful calming effect on the nervous system.
BERGAMOT *(Citrus bergamia)* **Antibacterial** **Antiseptic**	A member of the citrus family. The oil is extracted from the rind of the fruit and has a wonderful citrus smell. It is used in aromatherapy for the treatment of depression, amongst other things. Bergamot has a direct action on many strains of bacteria and is extremely useful as protection against all kinds of infectious diseases.
CINNAMON *(Cinnamomum zeylanicum)* **Antiviral** **Antibacterial** **Anti-toxic**	Must be used with caution. Its qualities have been extensively tested by the Pasteur Institute. Has a wonderfully charismatic aroma. Used against infectious diseases. Can be used as a disinfectant as well as an antiseptic. Anti-toxic, which means that it helps fight an overload of toxins in the system. It's very useful for many problems and is also a well-known aphrodisiac.
ITALIAN EVERLASTING *(Helichrysum angustifolium)* **Antibacterial** **Antiviral**	The flowers are often used in dried flower arrangements. Its strong, woody aroma is extremely pleasant. Very useful in treating mucus-like conditions of bacterial origin, it also promotes cell growth and in this way helps to rebuild a weak immune system.
LAVENDER *(Lavandula officinalis)* **Antibacterial** **Anti-toxic** **Anti-venom**	This oil helps numerous problems and has many medical applications. Curative and preventative. Used in the shower, its wonderful smell relaxes yet stimulates.
OREGANO *(Origanum vulgare)* **Antiviral** **Antibacterial** **Antifungal**	Better known for its use in Italian kitchens than for its antibacterial or antiviral properties. Nevertheless, *it is a very powerful oil* and must always be diluted before use. Oregano is highly antiseptic and along with thyme appears to have antifungal properties as well.
PALMA ROSA *(Cymbopogon martini)* **Antibacterial** **Antiviral**	Another anti-infection oil with a wide scope of action. It's good for both male and female genital infections and problems. A sweet-smelling grass, very agreeable and rather like rose, but it has a high level of bactericide activity. It also has a wonderful effect on the skin.
TEA TREE *(Melaleuca alternifolia)* **Antiviral** **Antibacterial** **Antifungal** **Anti-venom**	A relatively new essential oil. It's been extensively researched and is widely used in its native country, Australia. It has a stimulating effect on the whole system. It gives protection against snake and spider bites. A major anti-infection oil. It offers excellent protection possibilities.
THYME *(Thymus vulgaris)* *(Thymus linald)* **Antiviral** **Antibacterial** **Antifungal**	Thyme is a powerful agent that kills bacteria. It is thought to work by attacking the enzymes of the bacteria. Like many essential oils, it has a stimulating effect on the immune system. Its uses are numerous and it has been used throughout history for its antiseptic qualities. This is a very powerful essential oil and it *must* be used with great care – *never use it neat on the skin.*

synergistic formula for people who are at greater risk which is highly antiviral, antibacterial and antiseptic. Also, there are specific formulas for herpes and genital warts.

We begin with the massage formulas. These can be used for full-body massage, or a very simple and quick method, which can be most effective, is to massage the oil into the following areas: the armpits, buttocks, lower back, lower abdomen, upper thighs and along the top of the inner thighs by the hairline – but making absolutely sure to avoid the penis, scrotum, anus, perineum and vagina. There is nothing to gain by adding these areas into the protective essential oil massage, so just remember to avoid them.

You can use the massage oil once a day for a week and then when you feel it's needed; or simply if and when you feel you need to. If you have any allergies to skin cosmetics, soaps, perfumes, etc., it's advisable to do an allergy test on a small section of skin twenty-four hours before you plan to massage. As with all massage oils, make sure you don't get them on a condom.

Five Protective Body Massage Oil Formulas

Palma rosa	7 drops	Tea tree	10 drops	Oregano	5 drops
Bergamot	7 drops	Lemon	8 drops	Thyme	5 drops
Thyme	7 drops ◇	Cinnamon	2 drops ◇	Tea tree	10 drops
Lavender	7 drops	Oregano	5 drops	Bergamot	7 drops

Pine	5 drops		Patchouli	7 drops
Lavender	15 drops	◇	Lime	10 drops
Lemon	10 drops		Palma rosa	15 drops

Add to 30 ml of vegetable oil

One of the easiest methods of protecting yourself is by taking protective oil baths. Sponging under the shower is also quick and effective. You can use any single oil from the protective oils list, or the formulas below. Use four to six drops in a bath, and stay there for a minimum of ten minutes. Use four drops on a face-cloth or sponge in the shower following the general guidelines in the Method List on page 56. All the following formulas will offer you antibacterial and antiviral protection while disinfecting, cleaning and stimulating the body.

Six Protective Baths and Showers

Lemon		Pine		Lavender
Tea tree	◇	Niaouli	◇	Oregano

Grapefruit		Thyme
Italian everlasting	◇	Lime

Dermatect concentrate*

Mix each blend in equal parts: use 4 to 6 drops per shower or bath of any blend or blends.

Here is another bath or shower formula with the same protective qualities as the ones above, and using three instead of two ingredients. This is best made up into a synergistic blend.

Synergistic Blend
Bath or Shower Formula

Lavender	2 drops
Thyme	1 drop
Bergamot	2 drops

3-5 drops as required

*Dermatect is an aromatherapy product which is a formula of essential oils that can be used for infection of any sort. It can be used only in this section of the book.

If you already have a problem, a sitz bath is a more useful method of application. Use four drops of any single oil from the list of protective essential oils, or four drops of any of the formulas, closely following the directions on page 222. When using 'body-wipes', simply drop the essential oil on to a wet, warm sponge or face-cloth, squeeze well to disperse, and wipe the whole body.

Five Protective Wipes

Lemon	◇	Bergamot	◇	Tea tree
Thyme		Oregano		Cinnamon

Lavender	◇	Grapefruit
Palma rosa		Niaouli

1 drop of each blend

This next formula is a highly antiviral, antibacterial and antiseptic prophylactic. This should be used by people who are at risk, or feel that they are in danger of infection – in which case it should be used in conjunction with all other necessary precautions for safe sex. It also stimulates the activity of the immune system. It can be used every day if necessary – as directed – but try to save it for when it's really needed. It is a synergistic blend, which can be used in the bath, sitz bath, shower, or 'air patrol' methods. For massage oil, add the formula below to 30 ml of bland vegetable oil. A very simple and quick method, which can be most effective, is to use the 'super protection' massage oil by rubbing it into the following areas: the armpits, buttocks, lower back, lower abdomen, upper thighs and along the top of the inner thighs by the hairline – making absolutely sure to avoid the mucous membrane areas, i.e., the penis, scrotum, anus, perineum and vagina.

The Super-Protection Synergistic Blend

Oregano	3 drops
Palma rosa	3 drops
Thyme	4 drops
Tea tree	5 drops
Bergamot	2 drops

Prepare in a small bottle and use as needed

Airborne viruses and bacteria pose an invisible threat to the human organism. Protection can be offered against them by using the 'air patrol' methods for essential oils. This method has been shown by several investigators to be effective, including those at the Pasteur Institute in Paris who specifically tested the effects of cinnamon oil. They are an extremely pleasant way to offer protection at social gatherings. The simplest way is to place six drops of essential oil into a bowl of hot water, close the doors and windows and let the aroma waft around the room. One of the simplest 'air patrol' methods is to use a new plant spray – six drops to half a pint/280 ml of water. You can use any of the oils on the 'Protective essential oils' list in this section, or follow the suggestions for pleasant combinations below.

Three Antibacterial and Antiviral 'Air Patrols'

Lavender		Thyme		Cinnamon
Lemon	◇	Lemon	◇	Bergamot
Cinnamon		Lime		Thyme

The herpes simplex virus is a distressing condition that I have come across many times in my practice. It causes extreme discomfort and tiny blisters, which usually appear at the site of entry on any part of the body, as well as in the genital area. They usually come up between two and twelve days after infection. The following formula has been proved extremely helpful in numerous cases due to its antiviral action, as well as by reducing stress and anxiety which are often the cause of the virus re-emerging. Massage daily over the lower back, over the hips and the lower abdomen. Use for a minimum of twenty-eight days.

The Herpes Formula

Geranium	5 drops
Chamomile German	5 drops
Lavender	5 drops
Bergamot	5 drops
Oregano	3 drops

Dilute in 30 ml of vegetable oil

Genital warts are caused by yet another virus. They are small growths, usually grouped together and having the appearance of a cauliflower. They're found on the labia, the vagina, sometimes on the cervix, on the penis and around the anal area. Warts on the penis are called penile papillomata and must not be neglected as they can lead to cancer in the male and cervical cancer in the female partner. The following formula has been found to be very effective, but *it must not be used on the surrounding skin*, only on the wart itself. Keep the formula in a small bottle and apply it neat to the warts with a cottonwool bud (or use Dermatect – see note on page 224). It is far better to use too little than too much. Use once a day.

Genital Warts Formula

Lemon	4 drops
Patchouli	4 drops
Cinnamon	1 drop

It is vital to understand the dangers of untreated sexual disease and the protective and curative powers of essential oils have, perhaps, never been more needed than at the present time. The negative side of the sexual experience has already affected many unfortunate people, but with care you can do a great deal towards ensuring that this doesn't happen to you or your partner.

7

Ambience and the Aromantic Aura

Nothing is more important to humanity than love, and whether that love has been spiritual or emotional, it has always been closely associated with sweet-smelling aroma. In the excellent *History of Perfume*, Frances Kennet points out that most civilizations have made the association between sweet smells and 'goodness, friendly supernatural beings and immortality, and of evil smells with bad omens, malevolent gods and the force of death'. Today, sweet-smelling aromatic substances are an integral part of the spiritual ritual in many places of worship.

Nature's sweet-smelling aromas are not only an aesthetic delight to human beings, but bridges to our spiritual, emotional and physical interior, and in this chapter we shall be exploring a miscellany of ways to bring romance into our lives and to enliven love with nature's precious essential oils. You will discover that creating the Aromantic aura is very simple, and as delightful for you as it will be for your lover or guests. Aromantics are bringing right up to date a timeless human activity.

We are, indeed, very lucky to have access to such a

rich variety of essential oils. In times past the average man or woman would probably only gain access to the highly valued Aromantics when they were on the street – during the large state ceremonial occasions. These were extravagant Aromantic events. For example, we know that during the third century BC in Egypt, there was one procession in which one hundred and twenty children marched – all carrying incense, myrrh and saffron in golden basins. Behind them came the camels, each carrying three hundred pounds of frankincense, and others carrying the Ptolemies' personal supply of crocus (saffron), cassia, cinnamon and orris root. The King of Ancient Syria, Antiochus Epiphanes, was a great admirer of Aromantics and during his reign Aromantic processions were a way of life. We have record of one in which two hundred women walked, sprinkling everyone with 'perfumes', held in golden watering pots. In another, boys wearing purple tunics carried frankincense, myrrh and saffron in golden dishes. They were followed by two huge incense burners made of ivy-wood covered in gold, between which a large square altar was held high. We don't know if the Syrians – like the Egyptians – had braziers burning incense on street corners during public festivals.

The aristocrats of ancient time would have been invited to banquets at the palaces, where aroma was as important an element as the food. In Babylon, guests had their own individual cassolette, incense burner, at their place-setting. The aroma from this would have added to the aromas already present, which would have been considerable as the Babylonians were great consumers of aromantics. Herodotus tells us that they used to perfume their whole bodies with the costliest of scents. In *The Book of Perfumes*, Eugene Rimmel recounts a travelogue of Arabia by Neibuhr, in which the author mentions the habit of throwing rose water on visitors as a mark of honour: 'It is somewhat amusing to witness the discomfited and even angry look with which fore-igners are wont to receive these unexpected aspersions.

The censer is also generally brought in afterwards, and its fragrant smoke directed towards the beards and garments of the visitors, this ceremony being considered as a gentle hint that it is time to bring the visit to an end.' You should, however, consider it an honour if, travelling in Arab countries today, you are showered with rose water from the *gulabdan*, a narrow-spouted vessel designed expressly for this purpose. Had you travelled in Ancient Egypt you should have been prepared to be anointed in fragrant oils, and in times past 'anointing' usually meant letting the oils pour from your head to your feet! So it was when Antiochus Epiphanes, the King of Syria, bathed at the public baths and was approached by a man saying, 'You are a happy man, O king; you smell in the most costly manner.' The good-natured king immediately ordered a large ewer of thick unguent to be poured over the man's head. Unfortunately, a large crowd of people then tried to gather up what had been spilt on the ground, causing the king great amusement, until, in the slippery mêlée, he fell on his back in 'a most undignified manner'.

The ancient Greeks, who attributed sweet smells to divine origin, provide one of the most extravagant aroma stories in an account of a feast at which the host soaked four doves in different perfumes and sent them soaring above the heads of the guests, who got sprinkled as the birds were in flight. The Roman emperor Nero, who was an extravagant amongst an extravagant aroma-minded people, had a special ceiling built at his palace, the Golden House on the Esquiline, formed by ivory squares concealing silver pipes which could be moved from above to allow flowers and perfumes to fall gently upon the guests at dinner. Nero would not have been surprised to learn that similar contraptions, called 'aroma generation machines' are being used by Japanese businesses to stimulate the workers and relax the customers. Nero is reputed to have slept on a bed of rose petals and been fond of carpets of petals (a stylish touch he probably copied from Cleopatra's famous seduction of Mark Antony).

And for any fashionable Roman host or hostess, perfumed fountains were *de rigueur*.

King Edward VI of England (1547–1553) insisted on his rooms being suffused with the aroma of red roses, day and night. The method he employed was to place twelve spoonsful of red rose water and 'the weight of a sixpence of fine sugar' in a pan on the embers of a dying fire where the mixture would, apparently, scent the largest of England's royal rooms.

Queen Elizabeth I of England was equally concerned about making a good, aromatic impression upon her guests, going so far as to order a perfumed cannon to fire when she entertained the Duke of Anjou. This bizarre move would have been in addition to the usual aromatic additions to ambience – floors, walls and wall hangings sprayed with perfume. Like other Elizabethan ladies, Queen Elizabeth carried a pomander, either in her hand or in necklace form, as a protective against infection. Also, as was the custom of the day, she had a still room for preparing perfumes and healing remedies.

Napoleon Bonaparte and his mistress, Josephine, were both extremely involved in creating an Aromantic aura – her bedroom was thick with the aroma of musk while Napoleon preferred the aroma of rosemary. Amongst his belongings when he died on St Helena was a miscellany of perfume paraphernalia including an incense burner, reportedly used as he lay dying. An Aromantic until the end!

From earliest times people have not only sweetened their bodies with perfumed soaps, dusting powders, massage oils, deodorants and mouth fresheners, but also suffused their environments with scented braziers and room vaporizers, perfumed candles, clothes, cushions, pillows and bedlinen.

The Aromantic time is any time. Romance and courtship, of course, go hand in hand, and it's crucial to make the first occasion of lovemaking a specially romantic time, because that sets the pattern for the future. Aroma is a delight of creation, a bonus of life, and when you create your special ambience and

Aromantic aura, you join not only history's lovers, but also the alchemists, physicians, philosophers and poets of all time.

We start then with some room fragrances which evoke a variety of moods. The Japanese and Egyptians traditionally used a different aroma for every hour of the day: while that might seem like a lot of trouble to us hurried twentieth-century folk, the principle can be followed quite easily. You could start your day with 'Fresh'; then use 'Delicate', when your grandmother comes to visit; switch to one of the 'Tension relievers' when the children come home with a gang of friends at tea time, or after a frazzled day in the company boardroom. When you and your lover are together again in the evening, how about trying 'Relaxing and sensual', switching later on to – 'Passion'! The choice, Aromantics, is yours.

THE EVOCATIVE ROOM FRAGRANCES
SYNERGISTIC BLENDS

'Tension relievers'

Neroli	3 drops	Mandarine	2 drops
Orange	3 drops	Vanilla	1 drop
Pettigraine	3 drops	Lime	2 drops
Vetiver	2 drops	Geranium	3 drops
Lemon	3 drops	Bergamot	2 drops
Clary-sage	2 drops		
Lemongrass	2 drops		

'Sensual'		'Velvet nights'	
Rose Bulgar	5 drops	Jasmine	3 drops
Cinnamon	3 drops	Orange	2 drops

'Passion'

Jasmine	3 drops
Verbena	2 drops

'Romantic and sensual'

Verbena	5 drops
Hyacinth	2 drops
Rose Maroc	1 drop

'Innocence'

Lavender	3 drops
Tonka bean	3 drops
Geranium	3 drops

'Sensual and erotic'

Hyacinth	3 drops
Clary-sage	4 drops
Sandalwood	2 drops

'Caribbean – spicy and relaxing'

Pimento	3 drops
Nutmeg	1 drop
Ginger	1 drop

'Smooth island nights'

Bay	5 drops
Black pepper	2 drops
Benzoin	1 drop

'Passionate and arousing'

Lime	4 drops
Rose Maroc	2 drops
Vanilla	4 drops
Tonka bean	4 drops

'Sensual and woody'

Cypress	2 drops
Geranium	1 drop
Sandalwood	3 drops

'Romantic and erotic'

Jasmine	2 drops
Rose Maroc	2 drops
Chamomile Roman	1 drop

'Exotic No. 1'

Ylang-ylang	3 drops
Mandarine	2 drops
Black pepper	2 drops

'Eastern delight'

Patchouli	2 drops
Rose Maroc	2 drops
Sandalwood	2 drops

'Exotic and sensual'

Patchouli	2 drops
Verbena	1 drop
Jasmine	2 drops

'Hypnotic and heady'

Narcissus	2 drops
Jonquil	2 drops
Grapefruit	2 drops
Lemon	2 drops

'Arabian nights'

Lemon	1 drop
Patchouli	2 drops
Ylang-ylang	2 drops
Tonka bean	5 drops

'Relaxing and sensual'

Geranium	4 drops
Lemon	3 drops
Clary-sage	2 drops

'Fresh'

Vetiver	1 drop
Ginger	2 drops
Bergamot	4 drops

'Delicate'

Tonka bean	4 drops
Lemon	2 drops
Lavender	4 drops

'Masculine'

Cedarwood	2 drops
Bay	1 drop

'Opulent mystery'

Tonka bean	2 drops
Vanilla	2 drops
Benzoin	2 drops
Rose Maroc	2 drops

'Excitement'

Ylang-ylang	2 drops
Black pepper	4 drops

'Sensuality'

Jonquil	1 drop
Verbena	3 drops

'Masculine No. 2'

Mimosa	2 drops
Lemon	2 drops
Black pepper	1 drop

'Rich and heavy'

Tuberose	2 drops
Ylang-ylang	2 drops
Clary-sage	1 drop

'Caribbean'

Lime	3 drops
Nutmeg	2 drops
Tonka bean	4 drops

'Exotic No. 2'

Geranium	4 drops
Lemon	3 drops
Clary-sage	2 drops
Ylang-ylang	1 drop
Rose Maroc	2 drops

'Closeness'

Chamomile Roman	2 drops
Ylang-ylang	1 drop
Rose Maroc	1 drop

'Indian'

Benzoin	4 drops
Sandalwood	4 drops

BATHS

People take baths not only to clean themselves, but to relax and get away from the crowd. 'She's in the bath' is a distant echo we hear as the comforting warmth of the water envelops us, behind closed doors. This most special time can be made more precious still by applying Aromantic aura. Even the most utilitarian bathroom can be transformed by a few candles, a few essential oils and, if you're feeling romantic, a few rose petals floating on the water, illuminated by candlelight.

You can use any of the evocative room fragrances just listed if you're bathing alone, but if you're bathing with your partner I suggest you try 'Relaxing and sensual', 'Exotic' (1 and 2), 'Passionate and arousing' or 'Excitement'.

There is absolutely nothing new about luxuriating in bathtime. When Homer lived in Greece it was customary to offer a bath to the guests. But it was no ordinary bath. Here is an account of two men descending to bathe: 'Where a bright damsel train attends the guests; With liquid odours and embroider'd vests; Refreshed they wait them to the bower of state; Where circled with his peers Atrides sate.' For the Greeks, the power of aromatic baths was attested to by the myth that Medea turned old Eson into 'a perfect juvenile' by such an ablution. Knowing what we do about the rejuvenating properties of essential oils, this apparent miracle could be yours too! If your man is reluctant to indulge himself so, remind him of the Roman *thermae*. The largest public bath house that we have record of could accommodate 2,300 people, most of whom would have been men (women tended to bathe at home). Once undressed the bathers went to the unctuarium, where the perfumes and oils were kept. Here they were massaged before going through the cold, warm and hot baths. Only then were they given a rub with the best scented oils, ready to face the day, or night!

SCENTED NOTEPAPERS AND INKS

Napoleon Bonaparte knew that 'out of sight' didn't have to mean 'out of mind'. When he was away from Paris on one of his many campaigns to conquer Europe he wrote to his mistress, Josephine, on paper perfumed with violets. Men throughout history have received scented love letters and tucked them into their top pockets where the aroma could gently waft up and provide a constant reminder of their distant love. Just a little sniff would immediately bring back vivid memories of romantic times. We know that the Tudor Queen Elizabeth I used perfumed letters, not as far as we know for the purpose of keeping love alive, but perhaps to remind – through her perfume – the recipient of her formidable power!

Scent brings an extra dimension to a letter. Immediately, the perfume evokes memories of the sender and with couples today often separated by distance as they follow their individual careers in different towns, the art of the perfumed letter is needed just as much as ever.

Making Aromantic notepaper is very easy. Place four to six drops of your essential oil (chosen for the aroma your lover will associate with special times spent with you) on a piece of absorbent paper or material like blotting paper, tissue, cotton, linen or gauze. This need only be about 2 in x 2 in and when you've put the essential oil drops on this, cut it up into four equal pieces of one inch square. You can also use a cottonwool ball and pull it apart into four equal pieces – but not rayon wool as this doesn't absorb. Now place your four pieces of paper, material or cottonwool in different places between the sheets of paper in their box. Keep the box closed for at least twenty-four hours to allow the essential oil aroma to penetrate the paper, and envelopes too, if you like, in the box. This method gives a delicate scent to all the paper in the box.

For a more instant method simply put a drop of essential oil on a corner of the writing paper, where there isn't any writing as the essential oil could make the ink run. Seal the envelope and send. This method isn't quite so subtle, but it's just as effective!

Just as a couple may have their 'special tune', so too they can have an aroma which represents their unity to them both. And when one understands just how powerful and evocative aroma can be, this can be put to good use. Indeed, as well as reinforcing a happy relationship of the present, it's possible to recapture a lost love for the same reason – aroma evokes memory. Monika had been happily married for fifteen years when her husband suddenly decided to leave her and live with a younger woman he had met through business. Monika and their two children desperately wanted him back, but, as Monika herself admitted, 'I forever seemed to be busy chauffeuring the children back and forth and cooking meals at all times of the day to accommodate everyone. I suppose I never had the time to pay attention to myself or our relationship.' She felt that if she could only get through to him, everything would work out better now that she knew of the dangers of not paying him enough attention and making time for love. I had met Monika when she came to one of my talks, and afterwards she'd asked me whether I thought sending her husband a scented letter would ensure that he actually read it. 'No, I doubt it very much', I had told her. 'If he's in love and happy where he is, nothing is going to budge him.' Poor Monika looked pretty unhappy until I added the rejoinder, 'But how about using a perfume you used to wear when you were first married?' So Monika wrote her husband a letter on paper she had first sprayed with the perfume she had been using in the early years of their marriage. I waited to hear the results.

A couple of months later Monika phoned with the good news that her husband had returned home. 'He said he missed me!' she said, 'and had remembered the good times, the dramas and the love we had shared.' I thought that was the end of the story until five years later I met Monika again. Apparently, her husband had smelt her perfume in the flat he'd been sharing with his mistress and, sure enough, this had triggered the memories. He never mentioned the letter and neither did Monika, and it seems possible that the mistress had found the letter, read it as she walked around the flat and, perhaps recognizing that this aroma-packed letter could be dangerous to her, threw it away without telling him. We don't know (and nobody is concerned enough to find out). But what is certain is that her husband had recognized the familiar aroma – letter in his hand or not! (The moral of this story for mistresses: don't just throw the perfumed letter away – spray the house thoroughly, too, with your own 'special' perfume!).

The instant-recall of aroma can also be applied to writing inks. The staff at my local bank joke with me that they know when one of my cheques is in the pile they're processing because of the sweet aroma. (I always use perfumed inks!) This is another way of becoming a long-distance Aromantic, and extremely easy, too. Take any bottle of ink, any colour, and add two drops of essential oil per millilitre of ink. Most bottles of ink are 2 oz – so use sixty drops per bottle.

You don't have to use the most expensive essential oils, yet the faint fragrance will remain in the ink, and in the closed confine of the envelope the aroma concentrates and penetrates. When the letter is opened, a delightful aroma jumps out at the recipient – they'll know it's from you before they even see the handwriting!

Ylang-ylang leaves an exotic aroma on the paper, and while bergamot doesn't completely mask the inky smell, when it dries on the paper it leaves a delightfully fresh fragrance. Geranium is best for signing important contracts because it's all about fairness and balance – in this case, balancing out business affairs. Experiment until you find the essential oil/ink combination that suits you. (And reinforce the aroma next time you see your lover – in good situations only, remember!) As far as the recipient is concerned, there's nothing nicer than receiving a 'three-dimensional' letter – a combination of the word, the memory and the emotion!

LINGERIE

There's nothing so seductive as a half-dressed woman. Indeed, many men are more turned on by the sight of a woman wearing a few flimsy items of underclothing than they are by the nude form. Imagine, then, the impact of walking around in front of your man in lingerie and, as you pass, leaving a trail of delicate, suggestive perfume which stimulates his emotion and memory as well as his eyes!

People have been perfuming their clothes for at least two thousand years. The ancient Greek perfume expert, Theophrastus, gave complicated recipes for preparing perfumes that were to be used 'to impart a pleasant odour to clothes', and these involved a process different to that employed 'for bedding' (the Greeks were extremely fond of flowers and perfume and used them lavishly). In the sixteenth century, Venice was at the height of its trading power and the people perfumed just about everything that could be perfumed, including their clothes, shoes and socks. In Sicily today, the oldest and most widespread method of imparting a pleasant odour to clothes can still be seen when women hang the laundry to dry on rosemary bushes.

Making your lingerie Aromantic is even simpler than this. If hand washing, add two drops of essential oil to the final rinse water; if washing by machine, add three to five drops to the softener section of your machine. Alternatively, put the drops on to a piece of natural material and add this to your tumble dryer, as explained in 'Bedlinens'. Use a light essential oil, such as lavender or lemon, rather than the thick, resinous essential oils, such as myrrh, vetiver, hyacinth or mimosa.

It's also very easy to perfume your lingerie while it's in the drawer – and natural aromas are far superior to their chemical copies. Simply put six to eight drops of essential oil on to an absorbent piece of paper or material, about 2 in x 2 in, and then cut this into four and place these pieces throughout the contents of the drawer. You can make drawer liners, too – use blotting paper or an absorbent type of paper and add five drops of essential oil, one in the middle and four around the edges.

A young man I know, who won't mind me telling this story I'm sure, came to collect his usual oils one day and told me that he was madly in love with a beautiful photographer who was always travelling around the world to exotic locations with handsome male models. He was worried that she would forget him on her warm nights abroad and wanted me to make up a combination that would remind his girlfriend of him while she was away. I did indeed make him up a special mix of essential oils with instructions to spray the mixture around the room, especially before making love so that during lovemaking this special aroma would become associated inextricably with him – and love. Then, with this same mixture, he was to put a couple of drops on to a cottonwool ball and pop it into her suitcase when she packed so that the molecules could impregnate her clothing. He was surprised how effective a 'memory-jogger' this proved to be because on her next trip, his girlfriend called several times, without even knowing why she was calling. 'I just thought I'd call to say hello', she said, and even once called saying she'd dialled his number by mistake. By the ninth call in four days, she'd run out of things to say!

Any Aromantic can ensure a memory lives on. Add a couple of handkerchiefs for you and your lover to the scented rinse water with your lingerie, so you can both take one to work the day after a special evening of love to remind you both of what had been. Your workmates will never suspect that, instead of having a cold, you're reminding yourselves of sensual delights! If you wear a garter, imagine adding an erotic aroma to the swing before you throw it at him, and his delight as he catches your garter and breathes in deeply the Aromantic scent. As the French would say, 'Oooh, la la!'

BEDLINENS

When it comes to deciding on the aroma for your bedlinens, it's really a matter of personal choice. Five hundred years ago in England, lavender was a favourite and it seems to have stood the test of time well. In the seventeenth century, Isaak Walton was amongst those yearning for it: 'The linen looks white and smells of lavender and I long to be in a pair of sheets that smell so.' In the nineteenth century the English romantic poet, John Keats, mentions the favourite again in his poem, *The Eve of St Agnes*, '. . . and she slept azure lidded in blanched linen, smooth, lavender'd.'

The royalty of Europe had more exotic preferences. Tudor Queen Elizabeth I liked her bedlinen perfumed with sandalwood, while King Henry of France liked violet. In 1480 Edward IV was having his bed perfumed with anise and orris powder and, according to a document of 1633, Queen Elizabeth of Spain went for various aromas including rose leaves, clove flowers and coriander. At the most magnificent and luxurious palace of all time, Versailles, the Sun King himself, Louis XIV, indulged in a variety of aromas for his bedlinens. Ingredients included nutmeg and cloves, and there are complex recipes, for example, benzoin boiled in rose water combined with orange flowers, jasmine and a little musk. Louis XVI's wife, the extravagant and frivolous Marie Antoinette, had a liking for roses and violets until she met the French Revolution and the guillotine in 1793!

In days past, bedlinens were perfumed by combining them with little sachets of natural fragrance when storing or when laid on the bed. As 'Bullen's Bulwark' of 1562 records, they were also washed in 'a water of wonderous sweetness for the bedde whereby the whole place shall have a most pleasant scent'. History provides some complex recipes for perfuming bedlinen. If you were married to King Henry III of England in 1240, you'd be washing the sheets in violet-scented orris root powder, dried leaves of fragrant red roses, sandalwood, benjamin, storax, calamus root, cloves, ambergris, coriander and lavender. From the sound of it, you'd get both passion and sleep!

For Aromantics, things are simpler, and not only because we don't have to hand wash our linen! Simply add three to six drops of your chosen essential oil to the softener section of your washing machine. Alternatively, put three drops of essential oil on a piece of natural material and pop it into the tumble dryer along with the bedlinen. The rose essential oils have subtle, different influences on events – rose Bulgar is romantic and sensual, rose Maroc is heavy and passionate while Turkish rose is more gently erotic. You can use any single essential oil on its own, or make yourself an individually tailored blend from the information in different chapters of this book. Store your special blend in a separate bottle near the wash.

Total aroma bed kits were being sold by the eighteenth-century physician, James Graham, for 'couples desirous of child-bearing'. Above the bed was a special dome-like structure which gave off the smell of a whole variety of natural aromatics while the couple lay on a mattress stuffed with, amongst other things, stallions' hair, rose leaves and lavender flowers. The sheets, meanwhile, were perfumed with Tudor roses.

Of course we go to bed to sleep, too, and in England hops were generally used for this purpose. The fruit and leaves were stuffed in pillows and as the sedative effects of hops have been used for thousands of years, they may well have had the required effect (and not the same effect as when brewed into beer!). If you have trouble getting to sleep, I suggest you put a couple of drops of linden blossom or chamomile essential oil on a cottonwool ball and place it between the pillow and pillow case. A drop under the pillow can have a good effect, too, but of course in these instances the aroma is only confined to one area, whereas with perfumed bedlinen the effect is all over.

Natural essential oils can handle the heat of any washing machine; in fact they thrive on it. (Twentieth-century perfumes cannot be used because they contain chemicals which can have an unpredictable effect when heated.) Alternatively, put a drop of essential oil on a small piece of absorbent, natural material and then place this between the sheets in the airing cupboard. If you have a small, porous clay pot which you can hang in the airing cupboard, put a couple of drops of essential oil in it and leave it there.

Whichever method you use, or aroma you choose, nature's essential oils provide a truly delightful way of making bedtime Aromantic time. And as we spend so much of our time in bed, let's make the most of it!

CANDLES

No romantic scene is complete without candles. Their natural light and gentle warmth seem to diffuse a room with an atmosphere of delicate peace. At festive occasions all over the world the candles are brought out, too – the scented bayberry candle at Christmas in America being just one example. The traditional use of scented candles in places of worship probably stems from the very ancient and widespread belief that sweet aroma encourages the presence of the gods and drives away evil demons. The first Christian Emperor of Rome, Constantine the Great, provided aromatic candles for the first church of Christendom, St John in Lateran, with the command that they should be continuously burnt.

Many stores sell candle kits, to which you can simply add between thirty and sixty drops of essential oil per half a pound (225 gm) of wax – depending upon whether you want to create a gentle aroma or one with Aromantic force!

But you don't even have to go to the trouble of making your own candles – Aromantics can do it now. Take an ordinary candle, light the wick and wait until a little wax has melted, then very carefully place three drops of essential oil in the melted wax. After a few minutes a subtle fragrance will waft all through the room. If you do this with candle in a floating tablepiece, you could add a couple of drops to the water, too.

For a complete effect, when making or buying candles, one can even take into consideration the meaning of colours established by folklore over the ages:

Pink	=	love, affection, romance, gentleness
Red	=	sexuality, dynamism, stimulation, passion, vitality
White	=	purity, innocence, modesty
Blue	=	serenity, fidelity, devotion, sincerity
Green	=	fertility, tranquillity, calmness
Yellow	=	strength, happiness
Orange	=	warmth, cheerfulness
Violet	=	innocence, mystery

A floating tablepiece can be one of the most beautiful and romantic ways to incorporate all the power and meaning of fragrance, colour, candles and flowers. I don't think essential oils should be evident at dinner because their aroma masks that of the food someone has just spent a long time preparing (this didn't bother the ancient Greeks, who had perfumed lamps at their dinner table, alongside finger bowls with a lily floating in them). But after dinner, during a gathering of friends or when entertaining your lover, a specially designed floating tablepiece gives the ambience of the occasion a really delightful touch.

Find yourself a pretty bowl – a fluted flan dish looks attractive and can accommodate many blooms. Fill it with water, which can be coloured with food colouring if you want a total colour combination. To the water, add four drops of essential oil, then add the candles and, as the wax begins to melt, add one drop of essential oil to that, too. Now arrange the flower heads between the candles. Just one candle in the centre can be very effective.

A nice combination would be to take a white dish,

make the water pale pink, the candles white, and add pink roses and the exquisite aroma of rose Bulgar. According to folklore this would stand for purity and romantic love.

Or how about a white dish with blue water, white candles, with orange blossom floating on top and all fragranced with neroli essential oil. This arrangement could be taken to represent serenity and innocence. But for passion and sexuality, use red roses and red candles and rose Maroc essential oil.

Using candles in the creation of a special ambience and Aromantic aura can be as simple or as meaningful as you choose. Look through the various sections of this book to decide which essential oil to choose – there are those which relax or stimulate and those which reach through the limbic system into the libido! Or simply choose one of the evocative room-fragrance synergistic blends on pages 233–235. You can choose the colour of your candles and bowl-water by looking at the list on page 245 for the meaning of colour and – just to make sure you get the message across – follow 'La Code de L'Amour' on pages 251–253, which gives the traditional meaning of flowers in the language of love. You can experiment and create a total ambience decoration which will be absolutely perfect for any occasion.

LA CODE DE L'AMOUR

The secret code of flowers for lovers seems to have evolved in the harems of Turkey to facilitate communication between the closely guarded wives and concubines and their illicit lovers outside. It was introduced into England by the eighteenth-century poetess, Lady Wortley Montagu and into France by La Mortras, who shared exile with the Swedish King, Charles XII. The nineteenth-century lovers adopted it passionately, perhaps because romantic inaccessibility was such a feature of the times, with chaperones being as compulsory for these English ladies as it was for the ladies of the Turkish harem.

The language of flowers is a complex one, including negative messages as well as positive ones. For example, if you send someone narcissus it means that they are egoistic, and the African marigold 'tagetes' represents a vulgar mind! When you get a secret message like this, you can forget the Japanese saying, 'happiness is to hold flowers in both hands'!

The secret code was a two-way conversation with women sending messages to men as well as men sending messages to women. In Turkey women sent men flowers well into Victorian times, whether they were in a harem or not. When the code was introduced into Europe, it added to a long tradition of associating a particular flower or herb with a particular meaning – craftsmen already had reference books with illustrations of flowers and plants, alongside their symbolic meaning.

When Valentine cards were introduced during the Victorian period they would invariably depict a particular flower which represented the secret message the sender was trying to get across. A spray of rosemary was very often shown on the earliest Valentine cards because it had for many centuries represented the constancy of love despite being apart. Friends, as well as lovers, would give or send a spray of rosemary as a good luck talisman and, obviously recognizing the connection between aroma and memory, hopeful admirers would give a spray to their love to ensure the thought of them didn't go away! The whole idea is beautifully put in this 1584 sonnet by Thomas Robinson: 'Rosemary is for rememberberance, Between us day and night, Wishing that I might always have, You present in my sight.'

Many flowers have names which immediately tell their meaning in the language of flowers: forget-me-not, love-in-a-mist, love-in-a-tangle, and love-lies-bleeding. And everyone has turned to flowers to discover whether they are loved. Here, the poet Shelley tells us how: 'Full half an hour today, I tried my lot; With various flowers, and every one said; "She loves me – she loves me not".'

Of course, the colour of flowers has meaning too and, although we don't have space to examine this subject in detail, I would just say that red and white flowers in a bunch together mean death so, whatever you do, don't send anyone that combination.

All roses represent love but the red rose represents passion and beauty; the white rose means spiritual love and discretion while the pink rose represents simplicity and the musk rose, capricious beauty. The yellow rose traditionally represents infidelity, but only those who exchange the flowers will know whether it's the giver or receiver who's been unfaithful! If a man thinks his woman has been unfaithful but still loves her, he can give her yellow roses and if she understands the language of flowers and knows that he does too, she can take this sudden arrival of yellow roses as a sign that he knows, but still loves her. She may blush, and in so doing she lets him know that she knows he knows. And not a word has been said!

Roses have always been a symbol of extravagance and true devotion. It's said that Cleopatra spent half the wealth of Egypt to pay for a carpet of rose petals and other floral extravagances for a feast given in honour of her lover, Mark Antony. The Roman Emperor, Nero, must have admired Cleopatra's legendary style because when his wife, Poppaea, died the funerary arrangements consumed an amount of perfume and incense which was said to be ten times the annual Arabian output!

Particular flowers have always been used to mark special occasions. Aside from roses, St Valentine's Day is traditionally symbolized by the crocus because that is the flower of St Valentine, the patron saint of lovers. This may have something to do with the fact that 14 February is around the time that crocus flowers bloom - in Britain at least – or it may stem from the ancient Greek tradition of giving crocuses at the marriage feast. This, in turn, stems from the Greek myth: a beautiful young man called Crocus fell deeply in love with a shepherdess called Smilax, but she didn't return his love. The gods felt sorry for him and, to put him out of his misery, turned him into a crocus and Smilax into a yew tree. If you have a yew tree in your garden, you now know what bulbs to plant underneath!

The bay laurel has also been associated with St Valentine's Day. In Tudor times the leaves were gilded and given by lovers to each other. Tradition has it that if you place a leaf under the pillow on St Valentine's night and dream of love, you'll be married within the year. When going to bed, appeal to the saint and chant: 'Saint Valentine be kind to me, In my dreams, let my true love see.' Try it! Burning bay leaves and twigs in a fire not only creates a marvellous aroma throughout the house but – so it is said – will bring back a lover that has left. Few of us today have open fires, but Aromantics can put a couple drops of bay essential oil in a bowl of hot water or on a candle on St Valentine's Day to see if that brings the lover back.

Gilding leaves and branches was quite a common practice in past centuries. In England, gilded branches of rosemary were tied with ribbons and given to wedding guests and bridesmaids, who also wore sprigs of it on the left arm to symbolize fidelity.

Flowers are a vital part of wedding day celebrations and over the ages, different flowers and herbs have come to represent different aspects of the union. Yarrow was included in the bride and bridesmaid's bouquets to ensure seven years' love. Some bouquets included a spray of rosemary for constancy, while a sprig of broom given to the bride acted as a fertility charm. Orange blossom at weddings traditionally signified the bride's chastity and, hopefully, her subsequent fertility.

Different countries have their own traditions. In Japan, the peony symbolizes many aspects of the relationship – pleasure, ardent lovemaking, fruitful marriage and prosperity. In France, honeysuckle is exchanged between lovers as a symbol of their union. In Italy, jasmine used to be made into head decorations by girls in Tuscany on their wedding day and to dream of jasmine is said to mean that one will soon be happily

249

married. (To ensure jasmine infuses your dreams, use 2-3 drops of jasmine essential oil in one of the room methods outlined in 'Blending or Mixing' or on a cottonwool ball between your pillow and pillow case!)

The partner's fidelity has been a worry for lovers all over the world and at all times as we can see from the many charms to achieve this. In Rumania, women tried to get their men to accept a sprig of sweet basil as this meant that he would love her for ever and no longer look elsewhere for romance. In Italy too, basil has represented love, which is perhaps why Italian house-wives saturate their tomato sauce and pasta with it! Again, in Italy, cumin seed was thought able to influence emotions and was secretly given to lovers to keep them faithful. In Germany, on the other hand, it was endive seeds that were thought to influence emotions and they were sold in little cloth sachets.

Because natural aromas most certainly do work on the emotions, it's quite possible that some of these ancient charms did work. However, some aspects of tradition are rather far-fetched. For example, accidentally treading on a lily was supposed to mean that your lover had been unfaithful when, more likely, you'd just been careless! And gauging the durability of love by how quickly or slowly a flower faded was a widespread practice, if also an inevitably disappointing one.

Perhaps the best approach to the subject of 'La Code de L'Amour' is to suffuse particular flowers with your own, personal meaning. You can build up a new language for yourselves and make your own symbol-ism. In any event, use flowers to build up a wealth of happy experiences and aromatic memories so that it can be drawn upon later, and brought back to vivid life, when things aren't so rosy!

'La code de l'amour'

The Language of Love in Flowers and Herbs

Acacia	Friendship, pure love
Almond	Indiscretion
Amaranth	Immortality, faith, fidelity
Anemone	Forsaken, abandonment, refusal
Angelica	Soaring thoughts
Asphodel	Regrets
Azalea	Passion
Balsam	Impatience
Basil	Love
Bay	Glory
Bluebell	Courtesy, humility
Borage	Courage, bluntness
Calendula	Happiness
Canterbury Bell	Constancy, recognition
Carnation	Has two meanings: in Britain it is taken to mean good luck and is often given at weddings; in France and parts of Europe, it can imply bad luck and is given at funerals
Cedarwood	Love
Chamomile	Humility, meekness, patience
Clove	Resignation
Columbine	Folly
Coriander	Hidden worth, merit
Cowslip	Adoration
Cumin	Fidelity
Daffodil	Self love
Dahlia	Instability
Daisy	Faithless with a face of innocence
Fennel	Flattery
Forget-me-not	Faithfulness
Foxglove	Insincerity
Gardenia	Secret love

Geranium	(generally) Deception (rose-scented) Preference (lemon-scented) Unexpected meeting
Hawthorn	Hope
Heart's Ease	Remember me
Heliotrope	Eternal love, devotion
Honeysuckle	Unity, devotion, generous love
Hops	Injustice
Hyacinth	Sports and play
Hyssop	Sacrifice
Iris	Message coming
Ivy	Fidelity, confiding love
Jasmine	(generally) Joy, happiness, passion (white) Amicability (yellow) Grace, elegance
Jonquil	Sexual desire
Larkspur	Infidelity
Lavender	Emblem of silent sweetness
Lemon Balm	Compassion, fidelity, a pleasantry
Lilac	New love
Lily	Purity
Lily of the Valley	Purity, happiness will return
London Pride	Frivolity
Maple	Reserve
Marigold	Adoration, constancy, endurance
(African) Tagetes	Vulgar mind
Marjoram	Happiness
Marvel of Peru	Timidity in love
Mignonette	Admiration of your qualities
Morning Glory	Affection
Musk Plant	Weakness
Myrtle	Love
Narcissus	Egoism, self-love
Orange Flower	Chastity, bridal fertility
Pansy	Thoughts of courtship and love
Parsley	Rejoice
Passion Flower	Faith
Peppermint	Wisdom

Periwinkle	Fond memories, enduring friendship
Pimpernel	Unexpected meeting will occur
Pink	Pure love
Rose	(generally) Love
	(red) Passion, beauty
	(pink) Simplicity
	(yellow) Infidelity
	(musk) Capricious beauty
Rosemary	Constancy of love, remembrance
Snowdrop	Hope
Speedwell	Fidelity
Star of Bethlehem	Purity
Stock	Lasting beauty
Sunflower	Fidelity, devotion
Sweet Briar	Purity
Sweet William	Happiness
Thyme	Spontaneous show of emotion
Tuberose	Dangerous sexual pleasures
Tulip	(generally) Ardent love, grandeur, declaration of love
	(yellow) Hopeless love
Verbena	Enchantment
Vervaine	Enchantment, pure affection
Violet	'I return your love', modesty, simplicity, fidelity
Violet Leaves	Fidelity
Wallflower	Fidelity in adversity

ARTIFICIAL FLOWERS

Silk flowers last much, much longer than the real thing and are sometimes so realistic that people can only tell the difference between them by touching the petals. Their main disadvantage is that they don't have a perfume or, as I discovered once in America, they have a perfume made of chemicals. The spray of roses I couldn't resist smelling on that occasion should have carried the surgeon general's health warning!

But if you make up your own Aromantic flowers, not only do they have a terrific natural aroma but a potent Aromantic force. You can make up a bouquet with the exact emotional effect you wish to create by choosing the essential oil from the emotional charts, either in the 'Aromantic man' or 'Aromantic woman' sections (depending on who's getting the bouquet), and matching the aroma up to the meaning of colour on page 245. Here are some suggestions for flower–essential oil combinations:

Colour	Flower	Essential Oil
Pink	Rose	Rose Bulgar
Red	Rose	Rose Maroc
Magenta	Rose	Turkish rose
White	Orange Blossom	Neroli
Pink or blue	Hyacinth	Hyacinth

For the really exotic varieties of silk flowers you can make up a unique fragrance, using your imagination. To make artificial flowers Aromantic, either put a single drop of the essential oil on each flower, or put the bunch of flowers in a box with a tissue or other absorbent material, on to which you have put three to six drops of essential oil, and wait for twenty-four hours. What could be nicer on Valentine's Day than to receive such a thoughtful, powerful and long-lasting token of love?

8

Sensual Food and Wine

The ancient Chinese appear to have been the first to perfume their wine. The Romans perfumed theirs with rose and myrtle while chicory (*Cichorium intybus*) was reserved for times when one wanted to produce fidelity in love. Sometimes a garland of scented flowers was worn and then placed in the goblet before toasting a friend. Of course, wine is in itself something of an aphrodisiac and many a glass has been proffered with more than bonhomie in mind! The Egyptians, Greeks and Romans all used wine for its aphrodisiac properties, saying quite correctly that it brings warmth to cold parts. Ginger, sage and angelica are amongst the perfumes that were added specifically for this purpose. Today, lime is one of the ingredients in *Coca-Cola*, *Pepsi-Cola* and *7-Up*. Another important ingredient in cola-type drinks is Cassia oil – a drop in lemon or limeade will produce a homemade cola. Cassia is, in fact, a close relative of cinnamon, and it's also produced from the bark of the tree (*Cinnamomum Cassia*). Vanilla has for many centuries been considered an aphrodisiac, which is why it appears in many famous perfumes. The erotic connection was recently confirmed by researchers in

Bonn, Germany. Perhaps we can now understand why the word 'vanilla' is derived from the Latin 'vagina'!

The word 'honeymoon' derives from the old Saxon honey wine potion that men drank for thirty days after their marriage to help them in their lovemaking. One cupful a day was enough, apparently, to help them through. Here is the Aromantic version.

All drop-quantities refer to essential oils.

Love Flip:

An egg-nog cocktail for two people.

Blend together: 1 egg yolk
1 glass red port
½ glass brandy
1 teaspoon sugar
1 drop of rose

Then add crushed ice. Serve in your most attractive wine glasses.

Honey Wine

Take one bottle of white wine
Add 1 tablespoon of liquid honey
Warm over a low fire
Add 1 drop of coriander
And 1 drop of nutmeg

This is a very special rosé. It relaxes and encourages . . . but very subtly. This is a wine that works particularly on the limbic portion of the brain.

Rosé Rose Wine

1 bottle of rosé wine – sweet or dry according to your taste
5 drops of rose
Leave for one day.

You won't find a ginseng root in your local 7–11 store, but they are quite easy to find in China-towns, health shops, or through the mail-order pages of health magazines.

East–West Aphrodisiac Wine

To a bottle of sweet dessert wine add:
4 drops of cinnamon
3 drops of vanilla
1 portion of ginseng root

Leave to infuse for seven days and then drink with your lover.

Aphrodite's nectar is a very simple wine to make and great fun to drink. It's really rather special and based on an ancient recipe. When you have made the wine, leave it to stand for three days and drink one glass after the midday meal. This is said to give you youthful beauty and voluptuousness with an increased sexual appetite.

Aphrodite's Nectar

To 1 bottle of wine – red or white according to taste – add:
2 drops of rosemary
2 drops of sage
4 drops of cinnamon
4 drops of orange
2 dessertspoons of sugar
1 small (liqueur) glass of rum

The next is a version of a wine in *Les Plantes Aphrodisiacs* by Gustave Mathieu.

Cinnamon Wine

To ½ bottle of Malaga wine add:
1 drop of cinnamon
4 drops of lemon

The following is a recipe that is so popular that it has been adapted more than once. It appears in a variety of herbals and aromatherapy books, from ancient to modern times. This is my version. It's a recipe for making a liqueur and needs eighteen days before it's ready to drink – but it's well worth the wait.

Perfect Love

To 1 bottle of vodka, kirsch or eau de vie *(or any other type of clear alcohol) add:*
5 drops of lemon
1 drop of clary-sage
1 drop of cinnamon
1 drop of mace
2 drops of vanilla
1 drop of coriander
Leave for nine days and then make a syrup by adding ½ pint/280 ml of water
1 lb/450 g sugar
Add the two together and blend well by hand.
Leave to stand for nine days.
Then add 1 wine glass of brandy.

Essential oils make great additives to all sorts of food and drink – from soups and stews to teas. Their aroma is better than the complete herb, and their purity gives everything a delicious clarity of taste. Unfortunately, there isn't room here to go into all the culinary possibilities of essential oils (as if such a thing were possible), so I shall limit myself to providing a few Aromantic answers to the cheeky question, 'What's for dessert, then?' However, here is a salad dressing which also doubles as a dip and which should provide you with an idea of the possibilities so you can experiment further on your own.

Avocado Salad Dressing

1 medium avocado	¼ teaspoon salt
1 tablespoon mayonnaise	1 teaspoon Worcestershire sauce
1 small onion	Dash of Tabasco (optional)
2 teaspoons honey	2 drops of lemon (or use lime,
⅛ teaspoon garlic powder	grapefruit or orange – to your
	taste)

Mix all the ingredients together in a blender until a fine purée is formed. Can also be used as a dip for carrots, celery sticks, green pepper strips and various potato chips.

So, to the desserts. Presentation is especially important if you are making an Aromantic event out of dinner. This first dish could be decorated with orange or lemon blossom and served in heart-shaped dishes. These things aren't always easy to get hold of, but you get the idea!

Orange Blossom (or Lemon Blossom) Crème

1 pint/560 ml of milk
2 tablespoons of sugar
2 egg yolks, well beaten
2 egg whites, well beaten
3 drops of orange (or lemon)

Scald the milk, add two tablespoons of sugar and the egg yolks. Stirring well, remove the pan from the heat and add the egg whites. Beat thoroughly, return to the heat and leave in a bain-marie, stirring all the time until the mixture thickens while adding the 3 drops of essential oil. Allow to cool before putting into dishes. Serve chilled.

It's very easy to incorporate essential oils into any dessert – simply add one drop of your chosen essential oil to cakes, sherbets, custards, jelly or sorbets. One drop is usually sufficient, but adjust to your taste. You can also make rose crème. The directions for this are the same as for the orange blossom crème above (substituting a rose essential oil), and this can look wonderful decorated with rose petals, in heart-shaped dishes.

Yoghurt Cheesecake

2 cups plain yoghurt
½ cup fructose (or sugar)
3 egg yolks, beaten
1½ tablespoons pastry flour
3 egg whites, beaten until stiff

⅛ teaspoon salt
4 drops of lemon (or orange or grapefruit)
½lb/225 g crushed digestive biscuits blended with 2 oz/50 g butter and used to line a pie dish

Add fructose (or sugar), egg yolks, flour and essential oil of lemon (or your choice) to the yoghurt and mix until blended. Add salt to beaten egg whites and fold into yoghurt mixture. Pour into the digestive-biscuit pie shell and bake at 350°F, 180°C, Gas Mark 4 for 30–40 minutes.

After night follows day, and breakfast. Here then are two morning-after spreads to enjoy together:

Rose Spread

Rose petals – a large quantity, rinsed thoroughly to remove any traces of pollution
6 drops of rose
Sugar – 3 times the weight of the rose petals
1 cup of rose water

Pound the sugar and the rose petals together; then add half the rose water. Simmer gently over a low heat until the sugar is dissolved and sticky. Add the remaining rose water and the drops of rose essential oil.

Use as a spread on bread and biscuits.

Rose Honey

4 oz/110 g rose petals
1 pint/560 ml of boiling water
6 drops of rose essential oil
1½ lbs/675 g good quality honey

Put the rose petals in the boiling water and boil for ten minutes. Leave in the water for a further ten minutes, strain and add the honey and the drops of essential oil. Stir well. Pack and seal.

St Valentine's Bon-Bons

1 cup honey
8 drops of lemon or orange

Cook the honey in a saucepan on low heat until a hard, brittle stage is reached. Test whether it's ready by dropping a small amount into a cup of cold water. If it goes hard, it's ready. If it's gooey, continue for a while. When ready, pour the entire contents on to a buttered baking tray. Butter your hands and as the outside edge of the candy cools, fold to centre and start stretching while still warm. Pull and fold the mixture until it becomes light and porous. Roll and twist into a long, thin shape and cut into pieces.

SUPPLIERS

The following company provides a mail-order service for essential oils, diffusers and other aroma associated products. They ask that a large self-addressed envelope be sent when requesting a catalogue.
Essentially Yours, PO Box 38, Romford RM1 2DN

Australia:
Aroma Aromatherapy Essential Oil Supplies, 790 Burke Road, Cam., Melbourne, Victoria (882–8322)
Auroma-Australian Botanical Products, 54 Stawell Street, Richmond, Melbourne, Victoria (428–4192)

Dietary supplements
Lamberts Dietary Products Ltd, 1 Lamberts Road, Tunbridge Wells TN2 3EQ (0892) 46488

WARNING

Not all natural plants or plant products are beneficial to health. Deadly nightshade can be poisonous and stinging nettles sting. The following essential oils should NOT be used under any circumstances.

Bitter almond	Rue
Boldo leaf	Sassafras
Calamus	Savin
Yellow Camphor	Southernwood
Horseradish	Tansy
Jaborandi leaf	Thuja
Mugwort	Wintergreen
Mustard	Wormseed
Pennyroyal	Wormwood

The material in this book is not meant to take the place of diagnosis and treatment by a qualified medical practitioner. All recommendations herein contained are believed to be effective, but since actual use of essential oils by others is beyond the author's control, no expressed or implied guarantee as to the effects of their use can be given nor liability taken.

BIBLIOGRAPHY

Bardeau, Fabrice *La Médecine Aromatique*. Editions Robert Laffont, Paris (1976)

Bernadet, Marcel *La Phyto-Aromathérapie Pratique*. Editions Dangles, St Jean de Braye (1983)

Biodisiac Institute *The Biodisiac Book*. Arlington Books, London (1981)

Chang, Jolan *The Tao of Love and Sex*. Wildwood House, London (1977)

Dogget, Mary *Her Book of Recipes*. (1682)

Garrison, Omar *Tantra: The Yoga of Sex*. Julian Press Inc., New York (1964)

Genders, Roy *Scented Flora of the World*. Robert Hale Ltd, London (1977)

Gerard, John *The Herbal*. Dover (1975)

Grieve, Maude (ed. Leyel, Mrs Carl F.) *A Modern Herbal*. Penguin, London (1979)

Hall, Klemme, Nienhaus, Holzminden *The H & R Book of Perfume* (4 vols). Johnson Publications Ltd, London (1985)

Hite, Shere *The Hite Report on Female Sexuality*. Collier Macmillan, London (1976)

Hite, Shere *The Hite Report on Male Sexuality*. Alfred A. Knopf, New York (1981)

Johns, Catherine *Sex or Symbol*. British Museum Publications Ltd, London (1982)

Kaplan, Helen Singer MD Ph.D. *The New Sex Therapy*. Baillière Tindall, London (1974)

Kennett, Frances *History of Perfume*. Harrap, London (1975)

Kitzinger, Sheila *Woman's Experience of Sex*. Dorling Kindersley, London (1983)

Lavabre, Marcel *Aromatherapy Workbook*. The Healing Arts Press, Vermont (1990)

Maple, Eric *The Secret Lore of Plants and Flowers*. Robert Hale, London (1980)

Mathieu, Gustave *Les Plantes Aphrodisiaques*. Editions Sarl, Le Havre

Miller, Richard Alan *Magical and Ritual use of Aphrodisiacs*. Destiny Books, New York (1985)

Platt, Sir Hugh *Delights for Ladies* (1659)

Pratt, R. and Youngken *Pharmacognosy*, J. B. Lippincott Co., London (1951)

Rimmel *Book of Perfumes* (1865)

Rimmel *Rimmel Perfume Vaporizer* (1865)

Sagarin, Edward *The Science and Art of Perfumery*. McGraw–Hill, New York (1945)

Saxton Burr, Harold *Blueprint for Immortality*. Neville Spearman Ltd, London (1972)

Svendsen and Scheffer (eds) *Essential Oils and Aromatic Plants*. Martinus Nijhoff/Dr W. Junk Publishers, Dordrecht (1985)

Thompson, C. J. S. *The Mystery and Lure of Perfume*. John Lane, London (1927)

Tisserand, Robert *The Art of Aromatherapy*. C W Daniel, Saffron Walden (1977)

Tisserand, Robert *The Essential Oil Safety Data Manual*. Tisserand Aromatherapy Institute, Brighton (1988)

Trager, James *Letters From Sachiko*. Sphere Books, London (1984)

Valnet, Dr Jean *Aromatherapie*. Librairie Maloine, Paris (1980)

Drs Valnet, Duraffourd and Lapraz *Phytothérapie et Aromathérapie*. Presse de la Renaissance, Paris (1978)

van Toller, Steve and Dodds, George H. *Perfumery, the Psychology and Biology of Fragrance*. Chapman and Hall, London (1988)

Vatsyayana, (trans. R. F. Burton and F. F. Arbuthnot) *Kama Sutra*. Unwin, London (1982)

Watts, Martin *Plant Aromatics*. Martin Watts, Whitham (1992)

Winter, R. *The Smell Book: Scents, Sex and Society*. J. B. Lippincott Co., Philadelphia, PA (1976)

Worwood, Valerie Ann, *The Fragrant Pharmacy*. Bantam Books, London (1991)

Index

268

Valerie Ann Worwood is internationally acknowledged as one of the world's leading aromatherapists and is the author of the bestselling *Fragrant Pharmacy* and *Fragrant Mind*. Awarded a Doctorate in 1990, she has served on the executive councils of the International Federation of Aromatherapists and The Aromatherapy Organisations Council, and has initiated research projects into the clinical use of essential oils.

THE FRAGRANT PHARMACY
by Valerie Ann Worwood

The Fragrant Pharmacy opens the way to a whole world of fresh possibilities. It is a new approach to nature through one of its most powerful forms – those fragrant 'essential oils' drawn from flowers and grasses, trees and roots, leaves and fruit, that remain the great untapped resources of our planet.

The Fragrant Pharmacy shows how each essential oil can offer many diverse benefits. One of the most holistic of all systems of medicine, the oils can alleviate symptoms, prevent many illnesses and disorders and help in their healing process. But more than that, they can provide all of us – our families, our homes, even our pets – with the protections and pleasures we need . . . without the chemical pollution of our bodies or our environment.

This illuminating and imaginative book of aromatherapy is the household manual of the future. It is a treasury of information about precious life- and health-enhancing liquids that work in complex harmony with people and planet alike. Here is a comprehensive encyclopaedia of 'medicines out of the earth', those miracles of creation which revitalize and rejuvenate, enhance our emotions and help our work and play. It charts out for all of us a fragrant way to family health and home delights.

'An excellent encyclopaedia for use in everyday life'
City Limits

Available in Bantam Paperback

0553 40397 4